French Women Don't Get Facelifts

AGING WITH ATTITUDE

MIREILLE GUILIANO

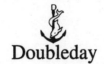

Doubleday

LONDON · TORONTO · SYDNEY · AUCKLAND · JOHANNESBURG

TRANSWORLD PUBLISHERS
61–63 Uxbridge Road, London W5 5SA
A Random House Group Company
www.transworldbooks.co.uk

First published in the United States
in 2013 by Grand Central Life & Style
an imprint of the Hachette Book Group

First published in Great Britain
in 2014 by Doubleday
an imprint of Transworld Publishers

A CIP catalogue record for this book
is available from the British Library.

ISBNs 9780857521484

Addresses for Random House Group Ltd companies outside the UK
can be found at: www.randomhouse.co.uk
The Random House Group Ltd Reg. No. 954009

The Random House Group Limited supports the Forest Stewardship
Council® (FSC®), the leading international forest-certification organisation.
Our books carrying the FSC label are printed on FSC®-certified paper.
FSC is the only forest-certification scheme supported by the leading
environmental organisations, including Greenpeace. Our paper procurement
policy can be found at www.randomhouse.co.uk/environment

Typeset in Bembo
Printed and bound in Great Britain by
Clays Ltd, Bungay, Suffolk

2 4 6 8 10 9 7 5 3 1

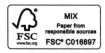

Personne n'est jeune après quarante ans mais on peut être irrésistible à tout âge.

No one is young after forty, but one can be irresistible at any age.

Coco Chanel (1883–1971)

CONTENTS

*French Women
Don't Get Facelifts*

AGING WITH ATTITUDE

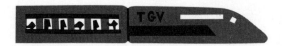

Last summer, my boyfriend in Provence—he is a handsome, dynamic, whirlwind of a three-and-a-half-year-old gamin, half French, half Indian—said to me, "You're old." "Yes, I am," I said. What else could I say? Of course, to a child someone forty is old. His father was shocked and apologized, but having reached my sixties, I've looked in the mirror. I now buy senior citizen tickets on France's TGV train. But I still travel fast.

The thing is, though, inside my head I don't feel old. I don't really think about age, though I feel it sometimes . . . and see it. In my mind, I am sort of ageless or at least the age in which I place myself in memory's pictures. Indeed, looking at old photos, I am a time traveler, fooling time and living inside those photos in the present tense.

Traveling on the TGV, though, I realize that I am as happy as I've ever been. And that's a surprise. People dread getting old or feeling old, but old today is ninety, not sixty or even seventy. But again, I am not alone in discovering that there are a lot of positives about aging. Here I am like the French women of my birth. As a class we are the happiest between sixty-five and seventy. Go figure. Works for me. Experts explain that it has to do with our maturity, which helps us make the choices that are good for us or satisfy us with what we have, whether we are women or men. Certainly at that age we are far less about becoming than being. We are not aspiring for a different professional position or career, our social set is well established, and we have come to accept our likes and limitations. And we don't have to deal with periods and PMS.

In America, I live in a youth-obsessed culture and a results-oriented culture. So old age is often cast in a negative light. We're less proficient at multitasking and don't look as good doing it. Is that a negative? I have a ninety-four-year-old friend who sometimes says to me, "Getting old stinks." Ah, but some people say that about being a teenager. I am always motivated by the very old to think about *what I can do* now to be better prepared to enjoy the next stages of my life. Economists to sociologists to psychologists try to determine the factors of being *satisfaits*, a milder form of "happy" the French prefer to show. I was surprised to learn that studies reveal we are the least happy between twenty and fifty, with possibly those forty-five to fifty hitting the least happy period and then increasing our *satisfaits* into our seventies. So be sure to celebrate your fiftieth birthday. It marks a new beginning to happiness.

When I was in my thirties and forties, I did not think about getting or being old. I mostly lived in the present, being busy and trying to live life to the fullest. I did, however, pay attention to living a healthy lifestyle. And in my four books on the subject, three with an emphasis on developing a good relationship with food and with yourself, I shared some of the lessons I had learned along the way. But they are only a part of the *art and joie de vivre.*

I have the genes to live a great many years, and I want to know how to attack aging so to enjoy it to the fullest. And I know I am not alone. My friend never dreamed she would live to age ninety-four and never prepared for the later stages in life the way I will. I am not thinking so much about living long, but rather about looking good and feeling healthy in the decades ahead.

Our world is graying: Europe is aging, America is aging, China and other nations are aging. I am a baby boomer, and a reality is that every day more than seven thousand Americans turn sixty-five. By 2030, 18 percent of Americans will be senior citizens, up from 12 percent today. That trend is true for the majority of nations. By 2025, one-third of all Japanese will be sixty-five or older.

Because of the reception of my lifestyle books and perhaps because I was born French, I am often asked to share my tips on "aging gracefully," an expression I don't like. "Aging with attitude" is what I believe in.

As someone with a foot in two countries, my native France and adopted America, as well as continuing stops all over the globe, I can sometimes see the advantages (and follies) of each culture sharply and share what seems to work well—and not so well—with other women. Take facelifts and other cosmetic surgery.

Cosmetic surgery all over the world is becoming almost a religion, and many people worship at the doctor's office till they are stretched like a too-tight blouse and bear frozen smiles. France, a country devoted to female beauty and where women of a certain age are models of desire, elegance, and seductiveness, is not a land of facelifts, like South Korea or America, for instance. French women seek a more natural look and feel, opting for creams and scrubs and, okay, perhaps a few partake in a little Botox or another filler, and look to what they eat and wear before the surgeon's scalpel. And when they seek a little medical magic, it tends to be liposuction.

Cosmetic surgery is not going away, of course; it is going to increase, and I am not going to fight windmills. Statistics show that Asians, for just one group, are in love with it. Just the way once we've learned to live with air-conditioning (87 percent of US households have it) and don't look to the off switch but to more efficiency and a wiser use of climate controls, the people of the world are not going to turn off cosmetic surgery, something that is more than four thousand years old. But it is not going to make us younger or prolong our lives. It is a part of the holistic picture for some people. I prefer to paint first from the inside out, not from the outside in, as a means for aging with attitude.

As one looks at the second half of one's life, it's good to have a plan, a strategy based on "knowing thyself," common sense, and a zest for life. For me, it is about being *bien dans sa peau* (comfortable in one's skin) through all episodes and stages in life. You and I don't have the same genetics, we don't live in the same places, we don't have the same resources, but we can have the same basic attitude: being comfortable in our skin. *Our own skin.* We are all unique, so no plan fits all sizes. Creating your own plan is vital, so you'll have to do some homework nobody can do for you. And a plan is a mental approach, an attitude.

The images touted in today's media, often of celebrities and then globalized, have made things worse. Yes, we live longer, but the cult of youth has made women more and more self-conscious and obsessed with looking younger than we are. Too often giving up seems like the easy way out. Too many women forty and up *se laissent aller,* let themselves go. Look around: fat is becoming scarily acceptable; so is dressing down, poorly, and distastefully (sometimes under the so-called umbrella of "comfort"). Then there are the quick fixes promoted on talk shows; in women's magazines and blogs; and with celebrities' recipes, tricks, and tips, invented by all sorts of "experts." American women tend, it seems to me, to behave in extremes; they are "all or nothing" in their approach to dieting, for instance, which I believe parallels how some women approach aging. They want and like to see themselves as young and perfect, but then they cannot ignore the slippery slope to getting old. Once they feel old, many give up. Why is that? It is attitude. The psychological and emotional impact of state of mind has a huge impact on our "exteriors."

It seems like every week a new recipe, diet, or product is born to keep you young, skinny, or beautiful. Believable? For the most part, no. Develop a system with some rituals, some fun and spontaneity, some fine-tuning and reinvention as years go by—nothing drastic or painful; and the earlier you start the better, but let age forty be your latest start date. It's nature's starting signal for sure. If you are past forty, no worries, but hurry up and hop aboard.

What follows is a multifaceted approach to attacking aging from forty onward so you will appreciate life to its fullest through your second set of decades. Age fifty? Certainly time to tune in. In fact, it's never too late to learn and share these secrets. What's helpful and positive is emphasized throughout, and the volume is rich with information and new tips and tricks to achieve a personal winning formula. As is my style, I have included stories and anecdotes from my life that I hope you will enjoy and that will communicate meaningful advice. The fountain of youth cannot fit between the covers of a book, nor can the levels of detail on any rich subject searchable on the Internet. However, an attitude and categorical approach can. This book is designed to assist the readers—women but broadly applicable to men as well—to devise their own formula for life that enhances their looks, health, and pleasures, and helps them be comfortable in their skin at any age. This is a call to take up arms against the onslaught of aging. It provides the keys to taking off ten years from your body and mind.

Now, as we say in French, *attaquons.*

1

ASSESSING GRAVITY

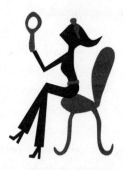

My husband has had a blond mustache his entire adult life. Except one day not too long ago he came to me and said, "You know, my mustache is all white." It is, and was, probably for about three years before he noticed.

I don't know what a fly thinks—if it thinks at all—when it sees itself in the mirror. But I know if we are going to manage our aging, when we grow older and look in the mirror we need to see ourselves as we truly are on the inside and the outside. A lot of us are kidding ourselves. We are not seeing the *now* us. We often are seeing who we *were*. Or we are blinded by who we want to be or who we think we are.

Truly knowing thyself is integral to aging well, being comfortable in your skin, and possessing a healthy, nondelusional, and uplifting attitude toward your own aging.

An essential element in aging with attitude is taking periodic hard looks at yourself in the mirror.

What should you look for? You cannot pick up a book or magazine or watch or listen to a program about aging without recognizing topics containing the "usual suspects": health, appearance, exercise, nutrition, lifestyle, medical miracles (a subcategory of which is supposedly cosmetic surgery), and relationships.

To which I want to add as a general category for self-assessment and eventually some self-modification:

■ attitude

Some of the specific questions you might ask yourself when looking in the mirror will come later. However, let's recognize from the start the power of attitude. It is a magic pill. And people have searched for magic anti-aging potions probably as long as there have been people.

FRENCH WOMEN'S ATTITUDE

Gravity works just the same in France as in the rest of the world, especially when you hit your sixties and seventies, if not sooner. But French women approach aging with a different mind-set than women from most cultures. With respect to growing old, the biggest difference between French women and most others is not grooming or clothing or nutrition or face and skin care; it is attitude. For starters, French women have a different definition of what constitutes being old. In a recent multinational survey, the French proved to be the least concerned about aging, and a cool third believed "old" starts *after* eighty.

Certainly in France, a woman in her forties and fifties is still alluring and seen as an object of desire and acts the part. She feels it and acts it, but doesn't pretend she is ageless. She is comfortable in herself. She takes care of herself and for the most part watches her weight and external presence, but she doesn't attempt to look like her twenty-year-old self. America and many other cultures are youth cultures. France is not. Name the top French actresses who come to mind. They probably all emote an air of grace and alluring beauty that is not picture-perfect or reflective of them in their teens or twenties. Juliette Binoche? Born in 1964. The still-iconic Catherine Deneuve? Born 1943. Even those in their late thirties, like Marion Cotillard, come across as "mature," exuding an alluring package of wholeness and experience.

There are a lot of young women in French films, but they are not endless Charlie's Angels, either. Consider goodhearted, flat-chested Amélie (Audrey Tautou). Women in their fifties and beyond are often shown as likely as not to have a lover, sometimes younger. While French women in movies and life may be petty bureaucrats in the office (a characteristic of the French) or objects of discrete desires, in their personal lives outside the silver screen, they revere being "intellectuals," both little and big. French women are able to quote the Rousseau and Descartes from their high school days and are ready to discuss and debate anything and everything, from the food on their plates to the merits of the latest political scandal. Being an adult is being grown up. And being grown up means losing some of life's insecurities, like worrying too much about gravity. There is much living in the moment for French women of a certain age, defiantly so.

You've heard the one that age fifty is the new forty. I have written that fifty-nine is sometimes the new sixty. Alas, there was a cartoon in the *New Yorker* that suggested, "Seventy-five isn't the new anything." Perhaps not, but it does suggest not holding back in your seventies...for what? Or even in your sixties and fifties *à la française*. *Carpe diem*.

FEELING GROOVY

How often have you heard the maxims "It's mind over matter," or "Stop thinking about it or it will make you sick," or "She lost her will to live"? They surely fall into the nothing-new-under-the-sun category.

What's new, however—if you consider fifty years still new—is we now have the scientific evidence that the magic not only works but is human science. The field even has a fancy name: psychoneuroimmunology. Belief is powerful medicine.

Remember the placebo effect? It's the fact that in many cases, the more a person believes in a treatment or drug, the more likely they will experience improved health or behavior. Placebos have helped reduce anxiety, pain, depression, and a host of disorders. A few decades ago it was scientifically proven that the immune system is connected to the brain, that there are complex communications among hormones and neurotransmitters.

Though hardly an all-in-one anti-aging pill, conscious belief and subliminal conditioning can control bodily processes, such as immune responses and the release of hormones. Put a Band-Aid on a child and somehow the child is soothed and feels better for no clear medical reason. We know a strong social network helps people survive cancer. Perhaps not a strict placebo but clear evidence of the brain's role in physical health and, obviously, associated mental health. Meditation, of course, is a mental means of ridding our minds of delusions and stress toward achieving a form of inner peace. Methods of meditation have enabled people to reduce blood pressure, alleviate pain, and effect changes in various brain and other bodily functions.

The point is, we have the power of making ourselves feel better. Let that sink in. It is a pretty amazing ability.

Realistically projecting, assessing the options, then shaping what we can and should be doing during the various later stages of life's road is the powerful mental medicine that can cure some of our ills and enhance our pleasures through life. Feeling groovy? Well, I do sometimes.

MEET EIGHTY-PLUS YVETTE

Growing up in eastern France, in Lorraine, I had a babysitter who over time practically became part of the family. In the summers, for example, I used to be packed off to my grandmother's country farmhouse in Alsace for a month or two, and Yvette did the packing and unpacking and ran daily interference for me with my stern grandmother...year after year. Yvette eventually married and had her own son and daughter to look after, and I left home for high school near Boston and college in Paris and a husband in New York, so we kept in touch mostly through my mother and an occasional cup of coffee. Despite that, we stayed close mentally. Eventually when my mother "retired" to the South of France, it was Yvette who could be counted on to check in on her and give reliable reports. And after her husband passed, she, too, "retired" to the South of France, in her case to the city of Toulon on the Riviera (home of the Airbus). It seems she found a wonderful companion and is living life in her eighties to the fullest with him. They even have a deluxe mobile home to go "camping" at a trailer park perhaps a half hour from their apartment. Every year now, they make a trip in summer up to my home in Provence for a much-anticipated visit.

Last summer, her delightful companion and her son, Claude, who lives in the extreme north of France, accompanied her. While we were having coffee with a piece of Tropézienne, the to-die-for cake named by Brigitte Bardot (yes, Yvette and I are both still very *gourmandes*, but now in moderation), the conversation led to New York as her son had come with his three daughters a few years ago and they had all fallen in love with the United States. Yvette said, "You know, Mireille, I am also here to talk about New York, as I really would love to come and visit you there to see the way you live." Then she added emphatically, "But I would like to do it *avant de vieillir* [before I age]." Now that was a statement from someone who is aging with attitude.

Right then and there we settled on the first week of November for a weeklong visit, displaying a live-life-with-pleasure-and-in-the-present-tense approach that comes with age. After she left, a thirty-two-year-old woman who was another houseguest said Yvette did not look her age but, more important, did not act her age. And it's true. Yvette has a pleasant way of meeting and looking at you, and her eyes alone project a light and conspiratorial twinkle that tell immediately that she loves life and is enjoying every second of it.

A few months later, I e-mailed her son to get some information in order to organize a visit she would love, and her son confirmed that she is indeed in very good shape, full of life and pep and curiosity, and maintains a good sense of humor. She eats everything, just in smaller portions than she once did, and while she could perhaps lose a few pounds, she is comfortable and healthy in her skin. What did she want to do besides see how I live? See a musical and an opera, he shared. Then a few weeks later she added a professional basketball game to her list. Perhaps there is something to the claim that Madison Square Garden is the world's most famous arena (and here I thought it was the Roman Colosseum). Physical limitations? I asked. She can walk fine, I was told, and the only thing she has problems with are stairs. *Hallelujah*. I reminded him that we have an elevator that goes to the fifteenth floor!

MEET JACK

Jack beat cancer. And he liked to fight gravity. I met Jack early in my public relations career in New York. He was our outside printer and would visit twice a week to work with me on various projects. I never asked his age, but he surely was in his seventies at the time, and acting forty. One day as he was telling me about his love of France, I felt comfortable asking what his "recipe" was for his optimism, energy, and vitality, not to mention his constant nice disposition and sense of humor. I learned then that he had a bout of cancer in his fifties that was life-changing. Things were not going well with his treatments in New York, and he journeyed into alternative medicine and medical treatments outside the United States. I remember Mexico was one of the stops. But what he found was a lifestyle and mental attitude that embraced yoga and holistic healthy eating. It was a long journey for this mostly bald, elfish man from his upbringing in Brooklyn.

What was his recipe? His reply was simple: "I do yoga every morning and particularly a headstand for twenty minutes . . . and I eat healthy." He saw my puzzled look, and before I knew it he was doing a headstand in my office to my open-jawed amazement. "Since my mid-fifties," he explained once he was right side up, "I eat less. I eat meat and fish once a week, and eat mostly grains, eggs, fruits and veggies, good bread, which I make every Saturday" (no Wonder Bread for Jack). "Baking relaxes me, and the most important is that I eat a lot of soups with lots of spices and herbs and yogurt" (the

French woman's staple par excellence), and which he made himself as he wouldn't buy the supermarket "crap" (his word). Granted, this was before some natural and well-made yogurts we have today. That said, we now have hundreds of yogurts that Jack and I would put in the junk-food category because they contain too much sugar, including in some dreadful corn syrup, often jammy sweet fruit, and preservatives.

I said to him that he was either Buddhist or French in his other life. He claimed a mix of both and claimed that since he had reached his mid-fifties and his cancer did not recur, he had never felt better. I often have the image of him in his business suit and tie doing his headstand, and I imagine what would have happened had someone walked into my office, and I crack up. I loved Jack and always looked forward to his visits.

Placebo effect for Jack? In part probably, but it works, and he had the will, the attitude, to live. And, of course, he hit upon yoga and a healthy diet, both of which were soon to be scientifically proven to facilitate a long life, which he enjoyed.

MEET DENISE

Admit it: we all know someone who we secretly wonder if they see what they really look like when they look in the mirror.

I have an old school chum, Denise, with whom I spent a lot of time in my twenties and early thirties. Now I see her perhaps once a year. And each time I am troubled and concerned by her appearance. Denise really needs to look objectively in the mirror. Don't we all? When it is not Halloween and we look like we are dressed in our Halloween costume, ah, well, it is time to ring the wake-up bell.

Sometimes I wonder: Should I make a recommendation to her about her hair or makeup? We have lots we can do to challenge our aging bodies and minds toward a healthier and happier march to the inevitable. I'd just have to figure out how to make a suggestion or two to her nicely. Or maybe she's actually happy with her appearance?

But alas, she does not seem happy. In fact, she seems to have "given up" for no reason I can discern.

Perhaps you've seen the signs of what I mean about "giving up." She wears only black, or very dark-colored, frumpy clothes. She has given up the discreet lipstick and eye shadow that were her accent lights. Her hairstyle is dated and not flattering. Seeing her conjures up an image in my mind of an old lady out of some European photo from the 1940s. I don't want to think that way, but I can't help it. And she is not old in the sense that she has decades of life left based upon her family history and genetics.

With each passing year I am saddened that the gulf between our "attitudes" is widening. I choose to approach aging with a positive attitude, with a sense of purpose and self-appreciation. Her attitude seems to be more along the lines of aging with apathy.

Am I being critical? Sure, yet realistic, to illustrate a bad case of not seeing oneself and not aging well with attitude. I've worked hard to create a positive mental approach to aging, and I want to protect that. When the women (and men) we surround ourselves with give up, it's depressing to be with them!

Can my old friend be shaken out of her lethargy? Just a few suggestions taken from chapters of this book would produce miraculous results. Maybe she will learn some secrets. But that would require her to see herself, and sometimes it is difficult for some women to face what's in the mirror.

Our female friendships are essential throughout our lives, but as we get older it's even more imperative to surround ourselves with positive people—people who have a similar outlook on life. Remember that old adage "You're only as old as you feel"? Surround yourself with people who are young at heart and take care of themselves, both body and mind...and watch what happens. I promise you'll like the results!

FORGET THE SPHINX

How do we help organize our thoughts and actions for aging with attitude? I say, forget the Riddle of the Sphinx, forget crawling, forget walking with a cane, forget classifying old age as the third age of man; it can be depressing and diverting. For the purposes of this book, here is the classification and organizational trilogy around which I approach aging with attitude from inside out: **mental**, **physical**, and **external** (*appearance* is one of those atypical nouns without an adjective form in English, but here I am thinking externally about the *persona*, the mask, we put on—the face we put on for the faces we meet). How do we look, appear to ourselves and others? How do we feel physically, our health scan and beyond? How do we think and feel mentally?

Naturally, the physical, mental, and exterior appearance elements of aging do not proceed in discrete linear fashion like infancy leading to adulthood. Often, they cannot be separated. Taking care of your skin yields a healthy skin and glow and a look that makes you feel good about yourself. Certainly being healthy affects your appearance and attitude and vice versa.

There are many questions we need to ask ourselves when we look in the mirror as we assess ourselves as we age ... from the general to the specific.

At the most general, ask yourself, *Do I like my appearance?* Are there things you can do to improve it? Do you want to? Some things like gravity are hard to change, though the effects can be tempered. How's your health? Are there things you can do to improve it? Do you want to? Read on. How's your attitude about yourself and aging? Are there things you can do to improve? Read on. There comes a time when you need to retire your bikini. Is it now? And how about those high heels? How about sex?

NEW YEAR, NEW YOU

Every year, as true as the sun rises in the east, comes January and major "New Year, New You" marketing campaigns for self-help programs. Health clubs offer special memberships and oversubscribe them because most people won't take advantage of the classes and machines in a couple of months. Miracle diet plans abound in magazines, books, and videos. Back-to-school, career-move ads and advice abound.

Certainly, the first of the year is a convenient and conventional time to make New Year's resolutions (of course, today or tomorrow is just as good for you to start your own twelve-month plan). The reality of resolutions made with the best intentions is that they are easily abandoned because the underlying plans are unrealistic and unsustainable. The yo-yo dieting that goes on each January, May to June (before the outdoor season), and the month before a big social event like a wedding is lamentable. Yes, it is possible and not that hard to lose five or even ten pounds in a month. Yo-yo...how likely is it that those pounds will stay off at the end of a year? Not very likely, which is why there is a new flavor of miracle diet promoted each January.

And that is why I believe wholeheartedly in *peu à peu* as the key to transformations. Changes that are drastic often don't stick. Taking things little by little means you arrive at your destination gradually, and if you fall off the path, it is easy to return to it. It's not failure but a slight delay. I also believe in taking an approach that emphasizes the positive, emphasizing what you can do, not what you cannot. Yes, you can eat chocolate and enjoy a glass of wine and not get fat.

A positive attitude adds good years to your life, but a positive attitude is not a plan for the second half of your life. Aging with attitude means an individualized plan for some mental, physical, and appearance adjustments for the upcoming year and with an eye on an extended horizon. While reading the rest of this book, if you can find even a half dozen ideas you can embrace and sustain for the coming year, you will succeed in adding good years to your life and hopefully more years as well. Okay, you might handle a few more, but don't pick too many to try all at once, or you will lose focus and fail more than you succeed. Hopefully some appealing ideas, both big and small, will just leap off the page at you. If you are like me and keep forgetting some items on the mental lists you keep, you might make a few written notes along the way. It is a beginning. Your first set of lifestyle changes will surely put you in a different healthy and holistic place in your anti-aging program, your aging with attitude program, a year from now and ready for the next look in the mirror and plan to defy gravity. Go for it.

2

DRESSING WITH STYLE AND ATTITUDE

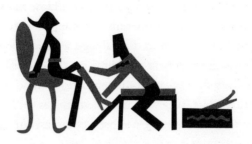

Quelle coquette! That's a nice compliment a woman can get from a man or a woman. It's a hard one to translate, as often in French the intonation can say a lot, but basically it signifies someone who is concerned about her appearance, a good thing, *bien sûr*; someone who has a knack for fashion, but who also desires to gain admiration, to please, play, flirt, or seduce, or all of the above depending upon the circumstances. When it's done a certain way—and to me it takes a woman at ease with herself and knowing herself—it shows. And forcing it also shows. Balzac said it best, "La coquetterie ne va bien qu'à une femme heureuse" (Being coquette suits only a happy woman).

Style, I have come to realize, is the manifestation of an attitude, and a personal style is a gestalt of many things, all of them about your attitude toward yourself and your surroundings.

Style goes with being *coquette* if we dress to impress. In France, the operative word is *seduction*, as social interactions for the entire nation have been and are built upon the art of seduction. And being *coquette* is part of the game. The French dress to seduce but not in the sense of attempting to lure one to bed (okay, not always in that sense). Plus it is something that French women would not think of abandoning in their advanced years, as it breathes life into them...into what they wear, what they say, what they think, and what they are. Look in the mirror. If you are not looking *coquette*, ask yourself why. Some of my friends would say, "Live, don't die."

At a point in my corporate career I had to make in-person, semiannual business result-and-forecast reports to Bernard Arnault, chairman of LVMH and now the richest person in France (some years the second richest). I vividly remember meeting him for the first time for one of these presentations.

He is quiet and reserved, though he can be cuttingly direct, and is known for his combination of engineering process and precision with his keen intelligence and heightened aesthetic sense, especially as relates to art, music, and style. He is also a French man.

When he greeted me for the first time, like a French man, he unabashedly looked me over in slow motion from the head down to the floor and from the floor back up to my head. It felt endless. "Il m'a déshabillée" (He undressed me) is the common French expression. *What is he thinking?*, I wondered. I'll never know, but I remember some of my silly insecurities coming to mind. *I am not wearing a Dior outfit*, I remember thinking (he owns Dior). I also was carrying a Bottega Veneta portfolio and not one from Louis Vuitton. Ouch. He shook my hand and said, "Bonjour, Madame Guiliano." *C'est tout.* That was all for the moment.

There is little question we judge people by their looks. Our looks make a powerful argument to a person about who we are. Clearly, Monsieur Arnault knew some things about me before our first meeting, certainly that my team was producing excellent results, but he did not know *me*.

What did my appearance say to him? What does it say to people I meet today on airplanes, in the market, at a party? What does your appearance say? It depends, of course, on how you present yourself in terms of what you wear and what your face and body project. And those are things you and I can control. It is all a matter of style.

OUR BIGGEST FEAR?

As we women grow older, arguably our biggest fear is losing our attractiveness, our very presence. We become concerned about our wrinkles, jiggly derrière, thinning hair, thickening waist, and, oh, sagging breasts. And it doesn't get better. Hearing aids are a cross to bear (though happily they are shrinking to invisibility), but we are shrinking an inch or two as well…and our posture becomes the dreaded crooked posture of an old lady. In short, we fear being seen as old.

The French attitude toward this fear is something like, "I see myself in the mirror for what I am. I accept that, and I am at peace with that; but I will do whatever is in my control to manage the message I send. And then I won't worry what people think. I will take care of myself and cultivate an image that is me at my current best and stay engaged in the world." That is at the core of French style and aging. It's an inbred attitude toward feeling good about how you look and looking like an individual set apart—that is, a person with a clear inner-and-outer style that is both comfortable to "wear" and distinguishing. And French women, if they are anything, are individualistic in how they present themselves. Their outer package is infused with inner style and beauty and an "I don't give a damn" posture (which half the time they don't, but they still dress to buy the morning's baguette).

Curiously, what I take to be an American attitude gone global is either a form of delusion—seeming to see the "old them" in the mirror—or an overly critical assessment of looking in the mirror and seeing every flaw. Some women tend to sit around and talk about nothing but how much they hate their thighs, their crow's-feet, their chins, their clothes, and how they are all wrong. It's almost a competition for who can be the harshest on themselves and point out the most flaws. Why is there nothing in the middle? We tend to lose acceptance for ourselves and revert either to lying to ourselves about how we really look or to self-deprecation. French women don't give a fig about perfection (and that applies not only to mix and match in their clothing but to many other aspects of their lives).

THE TELLS

When I was getting Monsieur Arnault's X-ray-like going-over, there is little doubt in my mind the two biggest "tells" of my "identity" were my hair and shoes. Did your mother teach you that, like mine did?

A great haircut goes a long way in making you look healthier, perhaps younger, and certainly more attractive. And dress however stylishly you think you are—upscale or not—and your shoes will still say it all. Expensive clothes with inappropriate or inexpensive shoes may send an unflattering message. (Less expensive clothes with good shoes, however, could pass as a style statement.)

In looking at your style and brand positioning as you age, shoes and hair are a good place to begin. Hair is about grooming, which will come later, but shoes...shoes. Shoes are key style signifiers. What is your style? What signifies your style? What sort of shoes do you wear? Birkenstocks? American tourists of a certain age can be spotted anywhere. Got an image? What's on their feet? I am all for comfort, but does comfort mean loss of attractiveness or identity? No, no, no. We have control over that and can achieve comfort and attractiveness and individual style.

Aren't high-heeled shoes sexy, seductive, sensual? They are in life and art. Are they for women of all ages? Let us consider the stiletto, epitome of seduction and sex. My friend Aurélie calls them "soft porn."

STYLE AND THE STILETTO

Certainly four-inch stiletto heels, made famous in Italian movies of the early 1950s (and now five-inch heels), make one feel and look taller and one's foot appear smaller. They are symbols of eroticism. People have fetishes for them. The wearer's posture is erect, bosom projected, calf muscles flexed, hips more prominent, and then there's the resulting walk.

But our bodies are not built for high heels. When should we elect to retire our heels? Our highest heels? Partly it depends on our balance and muscle tone, which we lose decade by decade. No point risking a fall (a fear as we age and lose balance and muscles and muscle tone). But let us not despair. My dance teacher friend Juju refers to stilettos as shoes women should wear *only* for sit-down dinners. The most stiletto-addicted woman I know can face the brave new world in them because she goes around by taxi or limo! Sitting down is the best revenge. Forget running down the street or dancing in them at any age. Wear them at parties that don't last through the night. Did you ever notice how we women of any age at parties and special events cannot wait to take high-heeled shoes off afterward or during? (Ever slipped yours off under the dining room table?) But we wear them nevertheless.

They make us feel young and sexy and pretty and different,

I suppose. Loulou, my stylish friend who just turned seventy and wears high heels to work daily, says she has worn high heels her entire adult life, so her feet have settled into them in a way that she is physically not comfortable in shoes without heels. Certainly she is not mentally comfortable without heels, they have become such a part of her brand and identity. What are your style signatures, and how do you retain and adapt them to passing years?

The shoes industry knows that too many of us can't resist shoes and works to provide us with a steady stream of designs that are fun and appealing. They feed the many friends I have around the globe who would be clinically defined as shoe addicts. Surely we all buy shoes we don't need; shoes that hurt our feet, backs, and posture, and sometimes break the bank.

We make many mistakes over and over, buying the wrong shoes for all sorts of reasons—feeding the fantasy of what we want to be, perhaps satisfying some psychological need or itch, satisfying an impulse (surely some of those *farfelu* impulse shoes send a message about who you are…the wrong message). We often don't think about which outfit we are going to wear the shoes with or even if we have something to wear them with. More often than not, the shoes are an end in themselves as opposed to what they should be: an accessory, a complement to what we wear, a personal-style definer, and, of course, a protective covering.

The key word for shoes, no matter if flats, pumps, or heels approaching stiletto, is *comfort*. (You might think "good luck" for the latter.) For me, wearing high heels is the exception, not the rule. I still have two pairs of three-and-a-half-inch high heels reserved for black-tie events or super-dressy parties, and although I've made plenty of mistakes buying shoes in my life, those two pairs were good investments and continue to serve me well and look new and trendy decades later. I have even danced in them without wobbling. One is Yves Saint Laurent and one is Bottega Veneta, both made in Italy and well made at that, which for me is rule #1. My feet apparently were born in Italy. (Indulge me...forget dollar signs for a moment.) These days my most comfortable ones are my black suede Ferragamo pumps, which feel like slippers and are my walking shoes in the city, on the plane, and more often than not at evening events. A few years ago in Amsterdam, I discovered United Nude, a less expensive brand (not inexpensive, though, *c'est dommage*) whose shoes are ultrastylish and ultracomfortable, including in what for me are high heels.

I appreciate that I have just mentioned some high-end, expensive brands, but they illustrate the French attitude toward a viable wardrobe: less is more. French men and women are culturally inclined to have fewer clothes "closets," but to fill them with quality and classics that serve them in many combinations over a considerable period of time. Adding a pair of shoes or one quality outfit is close to a zero-sum game. Something new comes in when something old is worn or styled out. Sure, over many years a French man or woman acquires and retains a "developed" wardrobe that has grown in size from the previous decade, but not all that much. Wearing out things and weeding out things not worn is part of the less-is-more approach.

Apropos, cheap and/or trendy shoes usually do look cheap and feel cheap. Invest wisely. Your shoes don't have to be high-priced Italian shoes. We all know a well-made shoe when we see it and wear it, and there are brands or off-brands or shoes on sale that measure up. I hear good things about a brand called Söfft and (who knew?) that J.Crew has a nice range of not-too-expensive women's shoes, including many manufactured in Italy. Then there are L. K. Bennett, Ecco, and Clarks for some good brands that are widely available at competitive prices. But whether cheap, moderately priced, or high-end, it all comes down to fit and comfort, regardless of how stylish. And if it were up to me, a class in learning to shop for shoes would be taught in school to avoid the trial and error of finding out what a "good fit" is.

I learned about "fit" after a reflexology session years ago that made my feet feel so good that I wanted to learn to do reflexology, so I bought a book and discovered that our feet can't be separated from body and mind. Call them the lower brain if you wish. If your feet hurt...(Hint, hint: just notice your tortured look when wearing the wrong heels.) It's similar to what the corset (nowadays the slimming shapewear) does to us when we want to squeeze into that dress (watch the red carpet at the Oscars to see the women who suffer... I would not want to be with them at midnight). Not the best options to look radiant.

What are we looking for in shoes besides the tempting design, especially after forty when physical changes reduce some tolerances? Try the following recipe: a mix of balance with good support and mobility. Plenty of seductive shoes offer just that when made by designers who understand anatomy, but let the final judge be you. And here's the checklist you did not get in school for deciding on investing in a tempting pair:

- Try both shoes, as our left and right feet were not created equal. (I've seen a countless number of women in a hurry just trying one foot.)
- Stand on a hard floor (versus carpet), and take a few steps to make sure the shoes are wide enough (always buy your shoes in the afternoon when you've retained a bit of fluid). The best test for a correct fitting is actually walking up and down a few stairs.
- Be aware that perfect sizing is impossible, as shoes are made from hardwood molds or plastic models, not your foot. I predict, though, that custom-made shoes fit to your feet will become more common in coming years. A sizing tip, though, is if the front line on the top of the shoe is higher up your foot, you will have stronger support for correct positioning.
- Look at yourself in a full-length mirror to check if you appear balanced, and make sure the weight of your body is equally distributed across the length of the shoe so that both the balls and heels are engaged for support.
- Don't let anybody tell you that a shoe needs to be broken in. Sure, a crease here and a spread there will add to comfort, but the wrong size will always be the wrong size.

MEET CATHERINE DENEUVE

If we look at photos of Coco Chanel, her clothes, shoes, and makeup all differed in subtle ways throughout the various stages of her life. I am reminded that we all need to "update" whenever I run across Catherine Deneuve in my Paris neighborhood, whether she's eating discreetly with a friend at a nontrendy bistro or walking down along the Jardin du Luxembourg or shopping in one of the small boutiques. She no longer wears stilettos or sharp red lipstick, and her clothes have changed, too, and so has her hair—shorter, freer, and her style is still elegant but more self-assured and timeless. Mind you, I used to see her and admired her already way back when I was a student and she was young and dating Marcello Mastroianni, who was living in the area. I'd see them walking hand in hand or sitting at the small but still-famous Café de la Mairie attended mostly by students and the area's intellectuals, and the picture was quite different: longer hair, thinner body, more makeup, higher heels, elegant style but very trendy, often in YSL. Today when you see Catherine Deneuve, you still can't help but go "Wow." She is a little rounder and not afraid to show her neck, which betrays more or less her age, but she seems to be saying comfortably, "Who cares? I am the whole package, not an aging neck." Part of her routine is a daily 5 p.m. *citron pressé*. She is an example of aging well and being *bien dans sa peau* with style and attitude.

BRANDING

I am a big advocate of being your own brand, wearing your own initials, not those you can buy at a luxury fashion store. Your brand is your identity, what sets you apart from others. It is what defines you and makes you memorable. Perhaps it is the scent you *always* wear that helps to define your brand. Perhaps it is a signature piece or type of clothing. It is hard for me to picture Yoko Ono without her wearing some variation of an old-fashioned newsboy's cap.

Through your decades you can evolve with the times without losing your established identity. You can refresh your brand without going for a complete makeover and attempting to become some new person. That's a bit like a crash diet, and such diets don't work. You will be back to your old self sooner rather than later. Better to tweak. *Update* does not mean "abandon."

Alice, my godmother, taught me about the "signature" element of the brand that is you. For her, it was all about her hats (and she did have a collection!), which she called the prolongation of herself. Being tall helped. She had a hat for every occasion and every season—for walks, church, market, for daytime and for evening, even for the garden—and with her hats she definitely turned men's heads around in a flattering way. A trip with her to the local milliner was an experience and an education. She would never leave the shop without a hat box. When I would tease her about a particular outfit, she'd say "C'est l'élégance du chapeau," to which her husband would reply, "No, it's because you have class, and it does not matter what you wear." They would *philosopher* (some may say argue) endlessly (a very French trait) about it. I came to understand that her class, style, and brand came from within (the "know thyself" that comes from looking in the mirror and being at peace with who you are inside and out). And for her, it exuded seduction and femininity.

As to "femininity," Alice was imperative: it comes and expresses naturally once you accept yourself. Adolescence works against us, and "becoming a woman is not so simple," but maturity and experience help. Remember Simone de Beauvoir's words, "On ne naît pas femme, on le devient" (One is not born a woman, one becomes one). A lifetime of ongoing inner search. Once we become a woman, it is not something we should surrender to age.

Jewelry is certainly a signature item for many women. While I believe less is more as you age, if you always wore frog charms on your collar or lapel, or a big diamond on your finger, why should you abandon them? What would that say? However, as your hair gets lighter and shorter in your "mature" years, those big pieces of costume jewelry or loops may need revisiting. Look in the mirror.

I suppose tattoos are a form of jewelry, though I have never quite understood permanently painting one's skin in heavy doses. Okay, a little ankle butterfly might be cute or some other symbol a form of individual branding. And while a new tattoo on a seasoned body may be seen as an attempt to be with it or recapture youth, tattoos have been around a lot longer than designer brands.

Pay close attention to your style and brand as you transition from decade to decade. What you wear and what it says is an exercise in attitude and expression. Enjoy cultivating your brand and helping it evolve with the passing years.

COQUETTERIE AND DRESSING WITH STYLE

Unless you are Sophia Loren, there comes a time when showing cleavage is a bad idea. For her it is a brand signature. For me, I don't have enough to matter, but I have mostly thrown away my bikinis and gone back to one-piece bathing suits. There's a phrase in American English that is very effective in describing an overexposed woman of a certain age plus five years: my cruel young friends would call it "gross." A more venial sin and concession to dressing our age relates to exposing our arms, especially our upper arms when they have lost a bit of muscle tone, and our biceps and triceps have a bit more jiggle than joie. Hold the sleeveless dresses and blouses! Learn to carry around scarves and wraps and long-sleeved sweaters. And while hems go up and down as part of fashion's refreshment and economics, it is the rare sixty- or seventy-year-old who can handle more than three inches above the knee. I don't want to see it, except perhaps on their daughter or granddaughter.

When I write about the French style of dressing, I am, of course, generalizing based on a core group of women and men who have traditional anchors in the past and have evolved over the last decades of their lives. This is the "Old"

France alive and healthy today, especially in the minds and hearts of the post-thirty-five set. However, fashion and style have become increasingly globalized and homogenized (and in France, multicultural), so not only do exceptions exist, but new tracks continue to emerge (in the "New" France), and some no doubt will lead to dead ends. But I am confident in mentioning such staples of French wardrobes as a good cardigan sweater in a neutral color. (Many girls in France grow up wearing uniforms to school, which surely carries over, including the obligatory cardigan as well as a less-is-more approach to wardrobes.) Other staples include, of course, a little black dress, a white blouse with high collar, a tailored jacket, well-cut and fitted pants, a stylish but comfortable travel outfit, a classic raincoat, and, *naturellement*, scarves and belts to accessorize and turn one outfit into three. It is the short list I revisit. The sexiness of your underwear is, well, your underwear. French women spend the most in the world annually on lingerie (but good, inexpensive basics for everyday wear). Oh, here's a tip: no one is going to be noticing your underwear's brand label. I cut mine off.

Business women, women of a certain age, and Hillary Clinton owe a huge debt to Yves Saint Laurent for inventing and popularizing the pantsuit as a viable fashion statement. Certainly a good-looking, well-fitting dress can be the most flattering piece of clothing a woman can wear, but a well-tailored dark pantsuit (or trouser suit, as it is called in many parts of the world) can be more than flattering at any age, besides giving great comfort, especially after fifty. It is the must piece for French women who like structured and polished clothes and a perfect combination for the twenty-first-century workplace. Wearing one well requires knowing your body so you can play with details from cut to shoulders to collar to width. Black (especially for evening wear), navy, gray, and maroon are the colors we still tend to favor, at least those among us who are pragmatic.

Often both a less expensive and more flexible alternative is the magic, timeless dark or colorful blazer over a deeper-colored pair of well-cut pants that make us look slimmer. French women like the idea as it gives us much more to fiddle with, starting with length and color. We love endless options. It's a bit like in cooking making three meals out of one. Effortless once you get the knack for it. We tend to favor tailored jackets that hit just below the butt. Pastel colors are great from spring to fall and give a soft touch to the overall look. My husband reminded me of that last spring as we were walking near our home in Paris and saw a woman—I'd guess in her late sixties or early seventies—from the neighborhood with a light soft-pink jacket and light purple pants that were striking. The designer Elie Saab used these shades in his collection, and it's all about refinement and understated elegance. Our Left Bank doyenne wore off-white loafers and carried a soft tote bag. She looked absolutely stunning. She wore it all with allure and elegance and projected a wonderful softness, and it complimented her age. Lots of classic women would rather opt for a shade of deep blue or Klein blue or emerald green as the one striking item, with the rest being in darker colors. It comes to picking what goes with the coloring of your hair and face, your overall look, and what you want to project. Know thy DNA.

When I retired from corporate life, I did not envision myself buying any or many dresses ever again, being partial to pantsuits. Then I was in Paris in November 2011 and walked by my current favorite designer's shop in the 6ème, Béatrice Ferrant, and saw a stunning dress in the window. I walked in and overheard the salesperson speaking with a customer to let her know that all was 40 percent off, as they were closing for good at the end of the year.

I've liked this designer for the substance of her line as well as a touch of romance. Her clothes can inspire while being elegant, well-made, and easy-to-wear couture clothes at ready-to-wear prices. I tried the simple plum-colored dress with a small leather belt and it fit perfectly. *I really don't need a dress*, I said to myself, but I could not pass it up. So I gave myself an early Christmas present (ah, how we rational-ize pleasing ourselves at times). A few months later, I wore the dress to a party in New York City, and I don't remem-ber getting so many compliments on clothes in a long time from women and men. I surprised my husband, who went "Wow" and said I should wear dresses more often. I admit the little dress suited me, and when you feel great in an outfit you know it. The compliments are just an added bonus.

As it turned out, the shop did not close, but rather just became "by appointment only." I recently arranged a long chat with Béatrice about fashion, trends, and what women should or should not wear. She is a delight, and is busy expanding to

China, where she claims there is a great need for dress code education and lots of businesswomen who love French fashion and are eager to learn. She is even eyeing America. I was thrilled. Here's a woman who is opinionated and knows how to dress women.

Béatrice's ideas come from her experience of working at top designer firms before establishing her own atelier, traveling extensively, and observing. She dresses women from age eighteen to eighty and has a lot of businesswomen in their late forties to sixties to whom she recommends avoiding black. That shocked me. Most of us should avoid it, she says. And here I was all in black. It may have been my only point of disagreement with her till she claimed that for me, black was one of my most flattering colors. Thank you. The transfer point is, if you feel good in black, keep wearing it. I agree with her that many women look older in black after a certain age. Perhaps in France there is an unconscious connection with widowed old ladies wearing black that influences us, though the mourning practice is a fading tradition. When my father passed away, my mother wore black only one day: at the funeral. She could not stand it and did not look good in it... "washed out" as she said. Who needs it? For Béatrice and many French women, including myself, navy, charcoal, eggplant, claret, and dark purple are the new black. Softer. Color gives life. Go for it, though pause before selecting orange or striking red after fifty.

Girlish looks for mature women are *not* something French women are keen on. With today's choices, one does not have to dress old at any age, but again, in France, a sense of respect in what we wear is part of the equation, which does not mean one can't make a statement or be noticed. Accessories are an easy alternative: cool sunglasses, a vintage scarf, an unusual belt or piece of jewelry on your jacket; we can all come up with some that suit us. My fashionista Parisian friend Mélanie, known among her friends as a frustrated fashion designer, still has fun in her late fifties playing with details like replacing the standard buttons of a dark blazer with pretty pearl buttons found at the Marché St. Pierre in Montmartre, or adding a lace collar to an old little black dress.

Textures and materials are important, too. French women generally favor what's soft, warm, and comfortable such as cotton, wool, flannel (some of us grew up with Damart flannel underwear!), jersey, velvet, and cashmere, as well as the new fabrics that make clothes affordable, casual, and cozy like the mixtures of cotton and cashmere, viscose and cashmere, silk and cotton.

Béatrice is opposed to jeans (vehemently so), and leggings as pants (except at home), overalls, any top that is shapeless (which, alas, is becoming more and more the norm as more women are overweight and think a loose, shapeless top hides their shape), running shoes, high platform shoes, and high boots. As I said, she has strong opinions. She was proud to describe how she dresses when she flies. Comfort, yes; casual/ sloppy, no. Not on a plane. Not in the street. Not anywhere. She loves pencil skirts, though not above the knee after fifty, and wears hers a bit loose to avoid tightness and let it flow; long cardigans over pants; belts are very effective to get a second outfit from a basic one; she loves dresses; she feels that investing in a nice coat with a flattering cut is a wise choice. Not the oversize kind that will soon be out of style, but a well-proportioned style. She creates clothes to reveal and not hide, and she likes to be looked at.

Coco Chanel said, "I can't understand how a woman can leave the house without fixing herself up a little, if only out of politeness." For my mother, it was a variation on the same theme with "You never know who you are going to meet."

I remember accompanying my mother on her Saturday afternoon chore of going to the cemetery to take some fresh flowers to the family graves. She would always go and change beforehand, though to me she already looked fine and clean, and it was, after all, just around the corner. No matter, she claimed dressing well was also a sign of respect, for yourself and for others. A sense of decorum is important. More often than not we ran into some important townspeople, and my mother's face would give me an *I told you so* look.

Still, style is hard to define—it is being your own brand, but it's born from a talent for living or joie de vivre; and it can be innate or unconscious, though you know it when you see it. It has to do with individuality (maybe this explains why French women are *individualistes invétérées*, or stubborn individualists, especially *les Parisiennes*), vivacity, passion, breeziness, enthusiasm, and curiosity.

For some women, all of this may sound trivial, considering that clothes exist only on the surface, yet this is not the same as being superficial. Clothes are, after all, about communication between a person and everyone who sees them. I see it more as just a basic human instinct, and a universal one for that matter. We all wear clothes and make choices about clothes, and nobody has any scruple about judging others' clothing.

My mother's idea for seduction and beauty and elegance or being chic was that they are all interrelated, and her motto was simple: "Be natural, keep your sense of humor, and do whatever it takes to be *bien dans ta peau* without torturing yourself." Beauty, like age, is an attitude. For me, elegance is also a silhouette, a look, a smile. When it exists, people will notice.

Diane Vreeland, the great Paris-born American fashion icon, said about style and elegance: "Style is everything... style is a way of life. Without it, you're nothing" (to which she added, "To have style you have to be born in Paris"). Well, that might help. As for elegance, Vreeland said, "The only real elegance is in the mind; if you've got that, the rest really comes from it. Elegance is innate. That's an attitude that works for any age. It is something to cling to."

Dressing with style, having style, knows no age and is a cocktail made with equal parts sensibility, personality, audacity (without going to the extreme), and some natural class. The latter is perhaps the hardest to get, though we all aspire to it. Isn't the best compliment a man can make about a woman "Quelle classe!" (What style!)? The best style is authentic, natural, and appears effortless. A woman may forget she has it, but when she gets noticed, she is reminded she has it.

3

SKIN CARE AND A NEW FACE

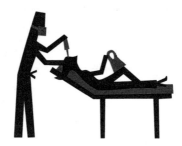

My Alsatian mother used to call it a "kaffeeklatsch," a sit-down with girlfriends over coffee for conversation, debate, and gossip. Never at one of these did she discuss the merits of Botox versus some anti-aging home-care trick such as argan oil, of that I am sure.

But as a sign of the times, I was involved in just such a coffee klatch last summer at our home in the South of France. And instead of coffee, four of us Frenchies were sipping various herb teas. Two Parisians and two adoptive New Yorkers. All girls (including the guy from New York!).

He had just turned fifty and arrived from Paris, where he had taken one of his "twice-a-year Botox sessions." He looks at it like getting a massage to feel better and tried to convince the three of us that we should go for it. "It's quick, convenient, affordable..." That philosophy applies more in New York than in France, even though some French women do Botox (none of the remaining three of us have, or are contemplating doing so, but you never know. I know I never would have imagined this conversation a decade ago).

We got into a heated discussion about the possible side effects, costs, repeat sessions, looks in between, needle effect (that's a turnoff); but also who to trust, as the best doctors are often busy dealing with celebrities, and the second-tier Botox givers are perhaps a bit iffy. Okay, perhaps if one has an asymmetrical facial problem or some cavernous crease, the upside of Botox is clearer, but for nature's little wrinkles? Have a treatment and start aging again the next minute and see the "old self" come back sooner rather than later? Oh, and how did we like that his forehead and whatever other part of his face he has Botoxed looks smooth and flawless, while the rest does not? Look at his neck... look at the back of his hands. There is something essential in the French mentality that is adverse to these methods: they tell the world that you have done something not natural, and that alone is a persuasive argument against most "miracle" interventions.

We all agreed that we would welcome softer wrinkles (unless we could have no wrinkles, naturally), but we wanted to keep our looks, our smiles, our facial expressions, and in one of those moments we shared a few tips, something French women are not always willing to do. Véronique used to be both a heavy smoker and a suntan-seeker till she reached forty-five and her skin began to betray her, showing the signs of her offenders. She is younger than two of us, but her face showed the most "wear." As a chef's wife and hostess of a grand hotel and restaurant, she had a stressful life that meant a pattern of two superhard months of work balanced with a week in the sun for R & R—not the best regimen, but her twenty-year schedule nevertheless. She is indeed looking for a miracle recipe.

Nadine had the best skin: she grew up with a Moroccan cousin who used argan oil as a beauty treatment, and for the past twenty years, she has followed her tip of a tiny drop on her face every night after her skin-cleansing ritual. It worked. Her face is luminous, her pores under control, and the skin is a tad oily, which is vital, especially after fifty.

Argan oil, which comes from the nuts of the argan tree grown mostly in Morocco, is exceptionally rich in natural vitamin E, as well as phenols and phenolic acid, carotenes, squalene, essential fatty acids, and some unsaturated fatty acids. The oil is increasingly available and is being increasingly used by cosmetic companies in anti-aging creams. Unfortunately, it is not cheap, as one tree produces just one liter of oil per year (though that bottle can go a long way).

So is argan oil Nadine's secret? Perhaps, but we'll never know how much of it is genes. She claims her younger sister looks older than her. She also does a few "beauty treatments" on a regular basis, from a chamomile facial steam to lemon juice washes and clay masks, all performed in the privacy of her home. She drinks lots of water, eats plenty of fruits and veggies, and walks everywhere. She is convinced her recipe works for her and sees the difference if she strays from it for a while. I'm convinced, too.

The last few years, she fine-tuned her routine, and to get a little booster added lupine oil in the morning. Yes, once again, another old home remedy revisited, as lupine oil is nothing new. Ovid used to say that after a night's sleep nothing beat a bit of lupine on your skin! I remember the lupine bushes in my mother's garden—gorgeous long-stemmed blue and white flowers, which I loved best after her rose garden. Apparently, labs have recently "rediscovered" the lupine flower's power as its proteins become nourishing lipids that hydrate while giving the skin a velvety sensation. Not bad. In addition, lupine proteins promote cell renewal and refresh the tone of the skin. A Japanese firm came up with a product based on lupine, and now several global brands are playing with the plant effectively.

Nadine belongs to the "know thyself" class of French women; she admits that she has tried a few "crazy" things and is now prepared for the next stage. "It's all about the three P's: prevention, planning, and preparation," she said. "Oh, and your energy, where do you get it?" asked Véronique. "Two-thirds is mental," was Nadine's reply. I am not so sure about that one. However, maintaining a can-do positive attitude, and executing a plan for mental, physical, and external adjustments, will kick up energy and appearance a notch... or two... or three. And Véronique? She is now using argan oil daily, albeit a little late.

What this says about the attitude of a great many French women is that they are all about trying their own routines, not emulating celebrities or buying creams that promise to "turn back the clock." They opt for natural, each to their own regimens.

French women do own a plethora of creams to work with, and, for some, looking around French pharmacies full of all these products is fun. The latest globalization of the French pharmacy is Sephora, a French company. Historically, French women seem to have taken better care and employ more pampering and maintenance to their skin than their global sisters. This component of the French regimen is an important export of the past twenty years. While creams will not remedy certain conditions the way some invasive medical procedures will, they are a part of a general spirit of maintenance, care, and pampering that produce positive effects. This practice is affixed, though, to expectations and goals not aimed at the extreme—and unnatural—results, but for preserving and caring for one's "exterior."

Some aggressive treatments, like a facelift, should be a late-stage curative, not a starter. Using argan oil, as Véronique does, falls into the category of all-important and underappreciated "preventives." Number one on the list is moisturizing in general. And for women in France, it is a religion. French women have been using the Nivea line forever, for example, the way Americans use the Vaseline line. Both brands are inexpensive but of reasonably high quality and fine for all body parts. (Don't skip days moisturizing your entire body.) So if savings or simplifying is a concern, these are good solutions.

SKIN CHANGES THROUGH DECADES

In the classic movie *The Graduate* (1967), young Benjamin, played by Dustin Hoffman, is uncertain of his future. An older friend of the family offers the tip "plastics," suggesting that the new technology is the key to a career and wealth and happiness in the new world. Then and now, the suggestion that "plastics" is the answer to important life questions is comic and ironic. When it comes to skin and aging, however, a single word is apt to the important question of why and how our skin ages and what we can do about it: *collagen*.

Collagen is the fibrous protein that constitutes more than 80 percent of our skin measured in dry weight. Starting in our mid-twenties, collagen production begins to slow. With the timing depending upon heredity conditions (outside our control) and nutrition and environmental conditions (within our control), wrinkles begin to appear and are noticeable by our forties. Most nonsurgical approaches to wrinkle reduction and looking younger relate to increasing collagen.

The other important element of our skin that impacts our looks is elastin, which, like collagen, is a structural protein. It makes up about 4 percent of the skin, and as its name suggests, provides its elasticity, letting skin snap back without leaving creases or wrinkles. As we age, our elastin loses its stretch and recoil magic. And over time it can become damaged, and the elastin fiber mesh network is replaced with less effective elastin.

Skin changes, especially on the face, neck, arms, and hands, are the most visible indicators of age and aging. They don't happen overnight; they build up under the skin for years, but by our mid-thirties, they are apparent.

In our mid-twenties and thirties, what we can look forward to is no secret: we get wrinkles, fine at first, but more pronounced later in life. The outer skin layer (epidermis) thins, which makes it more injury prone; and as our skin ages it repairs itself more slowly (wounds can take two to four times longer to heal). The color of the skin can become paler or even translucent as the number of pigment-containing cells (melanocytes) decreases and those remaining increase in number. So-called liver spots or age spots may appear. Due to both bone loss and thinning of the subcutaneous fat layer, we get sagging skin...and perhaps those notorious bags under the eyes. Sagging is the result of gravity. We see it all over our bodies with time, but it is our skin's loss of elasticity that leads in our fifties to visual sagging in the form of eyelids drooping, ears becoming elongated, and even noses starting to droop. And if that's not enough, as older people we pick up skin blemishes, tags, and even warts.

PREVENTIVES

While we cannot turn back the clock, we can make it run slow with good preventive measures. Let's round up the usual suspects. You know them. Look in the mirror and ask yourself if you need to redouble your efforts to apply those preventive measures rather than believe in an inevitable facelift or two or three to make up for not taking care of your skin before it became overly damaged.

Exposure to the sun's UV rays is by far the biggest contributor to the timing of aging, premature and natural. You know the horrors, including skin cancer, and you presumably know the drill. Stay out of midday sun, limit exposure, cover up, and use sunscreens. Sun exposure just hammers collagen proteins and connective tissues and makes the skin more rigid. Too much exposure and your skin can even become leathery and cracked, like a wizened old farmer's.

What is also within your control toward preventing premature skin aging is reducing your exposure to cigarettes and cigarette smoke; reducing your skin's exposure to air pollution; and keeping your skin moist, especially when subject to cold weather that dries it out. Naturally poor nutrition, lack of sleep, and overindulgence in alcohol are to be avoided. All show on your face.

The most basic and important routine to make your skin look and be healthy is to cleanse it. Don't go to bed without routinely cleansing your face to clean out and open up your pores. Soap can dry out your skin, so when you use it, be sure to moisturize afterward. Better to find a good cleanser or use the old standby, cold cream.

Periodically (as in weekly) scrubbing to exfoliate dead skin cells is a good practice. Exfoliating methods range from simply using hot water and a washcloth and rubbing briskly in a circular fashion to using a cosmetic scrub or mask available from just about every cosmetic company. (Men accomplish this simply by shaving with a good razor, though you would not think they know this by the flood of new face and beauty products aimed at men.)

Depending on your skin's oiliness, you will want to add some moisturizer after cleansing and especially after exfoliation. Don't clog your pores by overmoisturizing, though.

And not to be forgotten are nature's two best additives: water and a diet rich in vitamins A, C, B_3, and E. The last thing I do before going to bed and the first thing I do when I get up is drink a glass of water.

ANTI-AGING COSMETIC CARE

Whenever I fly from New York to Paris, which is often, I pass by the duty-free airport shops and see them jammed with Asians, including flight crews. The women all seem to be buying cosmetics and perfumes. It's not hard to figure out that the prices have to be much lower there than in their countries. Because the Air France terminal at JFK is home to the two biggest Chinese airlines, I found out many of these customers are Chinese. Such "luxury" products have high import taxes in China, thus the run on the duty-free shops in New York's JFK and the large number of Chinese-speaking sales reps who work the hours before departures to China.

What I also came to learn, and it was a surprise, was that the women were buying large amounts of the new age anti-aging products such as Estée Lauder's Advanced Night Repair (subtitled "Synchronized Recovery Complex/*Complexe de réparation synchronisée*) and described as a serum. Estée Lauder's Re-Nutriv line seemed to be a duty-free favorite as well.

Now Estée Lauder is a fine, reputable, and in this instance, representative company. I could have used Lancôme or any of several dozen brands, all now offering a range of semi-fountain-of-youth potions in a jar or bottle.

These anti-aging creams are expensive and require daily use for weeks to achieve their professed results in defeating sagging, wrinkling, coloring, or growths.

With the 40-plus million Americans older than age sixty-five due to increase to 88 million by 2050, this is certainly a growth segment for cosmetics companies. Considering that China currently has 200 million people over the age of sixty, and the world's population of over-sixties will reach 2 billion by 2050, we can clearly appreciate that addressing the aging population is a twenty-first-century phenomenon and a global business opportunity as well as an R & D (research and development) focus of the global cosmetics companies. The age of wrinkles is upon us.

Currently, these products are classed as cosmetics, as their medical effectiveness is yet unproven. By using words like *serum*, *DNA*, and even *laboratory*, these products are being disguised or presented as medicine-like.

I have little doubt that with all the investment that will be made in finding the most effective creams and liquids, some day they will constitute a proven class of effective "medicines," or at least treatments with proven results. I also have little doubt that most of what is on the market from reputable brands has some benefits, like reducing noticeable wrinkles by 5 to 10 percent. Estée Lauder claims that their Advanced Night Repair products have been tested and proved, and "88 percent of women said their skin looked smoother, more radiant, felt more hydrated." I believe them…and the women believe they look better. And thinking they look better is important medicine of a psychoneuroimmunological kind. As I wrote earlier, belief is powerful medicine.

Finally, I believe these anti-aging "serums" do no harm and probably do good, if at an inflated price. I have little doubt that proper cleansing, and utilizing a low-cost moisturizer and a sunscreen, currently provides the most fundamental anti-aging potion for all.

TREATMENTS

Being French, I am of the mind that every woman should have a "secret" treatment that provides her with an opportunity to pamper herself and gain results that make her feel more confident about herself. For some women, a "treatment" may mean a simple at-home remedy, such as a relaxing mask on a quiet night. (I like some rituals of this kind my mother taught me, even though there are commercial versions today that probably work as well or better. Do I use them out of respect? Nostalgia? Perhaps, but I use them first because they work.) Some people are into much more invasive treatments.

So it goes. However, I have realized that many women don't know what they're getting into, because the promised results just short of a magic fountain of youth of an over-abundance of beauty treatments are often misleading. Some women try every new treatment, spending hundreds if not thousands of dollars and never feeling good about themselves. Expectations are key, and we have to separate the psychological benefits of some of these over-the-counter creams, serums, and elixirs from their external results. But that is an individual question best asked in front of the mirror.

If you've ever felt overwhelmed by the amount of "beauty" treatments that exist... you're not alone. There's no shortage of options out there—most with technical-sounding names whose claims seem dubious (Can they *really* remove *all* my wrinkles?) or nebulous at best (What does a chemical peel *really* do?).

I do not claim to be an expert in beauty treatments, and I cannot speak of any of these from experience; however, I feel that women over forty should at least know what each of these treatments really does, as well as the benefits and risks associated with each before they spend the money or time on them.

Chemical Peels. "Chemical peel" is a broad term given to a handful of different types of treatments where a type of acid such as glycolic acid, trichloroacetic acid, salicylic acid, or carbolic acid (phenol) is applied to the face with the intent of "burning" the skin. This procedure actually destroys part of the skin in a controlled way so that new skin can grow in its place.

The type of acid that is applied determines the depth of the peel. Some acids are milder and remove only one layer of skin, often the dead skin cells only, but stronger acids go deeper into the epidermis and remove more skin. The latter, of course, come with more risk.

That risk can range from a slight burning sensation and

redness, to swelling, permanent color changes in the skin, and even scarring. And remember, all chemical peels create an increased sensitivity to sunlight.

Proponents of chemical peels report skin that is smoother and more evenly textured. Many women claim that chemical peels create a more radiant complexion and "younger"-looking skin—which makes sense if you think about the process. You're literally removing old skin and exposing new, younger skin that hasn't been weathered yet by environmental factors.

Microdermabrasion is a less invasive procedure that is essentially a professional exfoliation. A technician uses an abrasion tool to remove dead skin cells from the surface of the skin. The action also helps stimulate blood flow to the skin, which can reduce the appearance of wrinkles. The only risk is a bit of pain (the sensation has been described as sandpaper on the skin), redness, or skin sensitivity that typically fades within a few hours.

Photorejuvenation, also known as IPL (intense pulsed light treatment), uses light wavelengths to penetrate and correct color imbalances in the skin such as sunspots and age spots, blotches, rosacea, and broken blood vessels. Though it can improve the appearance of the skin overall, it's not recommended as a wrinkle treatment. There is little to no associated discomfort; however, IPL does carry a small risk of burning the skin if not done correctly. You will need three to five treatments, spread out between three and six weeks. The more sun damage or redness you have, the more treatments needed. Each session costs a few hundred dollars (depending on where you live), so multiple sessions can cost anywhere from $1,000 to $2,000! However, treatments can last from eighteen to twenty months.

And of course, the word on everyone's minds when it comes to treatments. The infamous *B* word...Botox.

Although it seems like it's been around forever, Botox was actually approved by the FDA in 2002, exploding like wildfire on the Hollywood and entertainment scene. It certainly made fifty the new forty.

Soon women from all across America were slipping into doctors' offices on the sly, and the phrase "looks good for her age" seemed to quadruple in the country's lexicon. Last year in the United States, there were more than 5.6 million recorded Botox procedures—and that number is growing by an additional 5 percent every year.

The reason why it's such a pervasive phenomenon is because, let's face it, it works! It *does* reduce wrinkles. Sometimes all too well, as it has become the fodder of "frozen face" jokes when many a woman (or man) has gone a bit too far with it!

Almost 82 percent of Botox patients report visible improvement within a week of treatment. But, like all good things, it doesn't last forever. And thus begins a cycle of consistently needing it to maintain the illusion.

Botox also comes with a considerable price tag (in New York, an average of $380 per treatment, possibly four times a year—treatments usually last three to four months—and that's just the first year).

As with any treatment, Botox comes with some risks,

such as pain and bruising at the injection site, headache, and temporary muscle weakness. And though it's very unlikely, it's possible to experience botulism-like signs and symptoms such as nausea, shortness of breath, body pain, and weakness.

But for me, I think the greatest risk would be that you can become dependent on a procedure that freezes your face in time. To me it's not aging with attitude, though perhaps with the bliss of ignorance. I wonder if the day will come when the absence of wrinkles will be the only way to spot old age.

So I say *non* to the needle. But you never know. I have a very smart friend who is a health and beauty writer and editor who uses Botox and advocates for it. Doubtful, though. I'll take a few wrinkles and spend my time and my money elsewhere.

We have almost reached the facelifts of the title discussion, but it should be clear by now that I believe there is an enormous number of things one can and should do before asking oneself the facelift question. I'm resigned to the reality that there always have been and probably always will be facelifts. And in some cases, I am a supporter. I completely understand that if you make your living with your face as a key contributor, such as a TV news anchor or an actor, there may come a time sooner than with others when you need to exploit the benefits of all science's tools toward staying employed. Men are increasingly joining women in preserving their appropriate look in the executive suite and beyond and in online photos. In magazines we already figure there's Photoshop retouching. In America, people seem to want to project youthfulness, while in France, people want to look comfortable in their skin and not tired.

ADDING A LITTLE HEAT

With so many baby boomers developing wrinkles daily (more people in this category are alive than all the people in the history of the world who ever lived and had wrinkles), there's a big market demanding new scientific antidotes as options to a scalpel or perhaps as a final phase before a facelift.

Certainly science, technology, and business will drive new medical options in the near future to counteract wrinkles and overt signs of aging. Medicine in general is changing rapidly, with discoveries and applications rewriting textbook remedies and procedures occurring at the fastest rate in history...and accelerating. We can't predict what tools will be in our medical kits in a decade. Fingers crossed. Science is at work.

Remember, the key word is *plastics*...I mean *collagen*. One new pre-facelift procedure that intrigues and is promising uses radio waves or ultrasound to increase the growth of collagen. Heat is applied to the face and voilà!; in one clinical trial study, 37 percent of the skin-tightening results of a conventional facelift were achieved. Perhaps here's a way to postpone the inevitable.

These variations of a warm massage—heating the skin with focused 104° to 150°F implements—produce minimal pain, and there is no need to stay out of sight while recovering. One or a series of treatments can result in providing a more youthful look and tighten up sagging jawlines and other lines.

Leading companies developing these procedures and their products include Solta Medical, Inc. (Thermage); Ellman International, Inc. (Pellevé); Ulthera, Inc. (Ultherapy); and Syneron Medical Ltd. (ReFirme).

According to the producer of Ultherapy, this procedure "can help turn back the signs of aging by noninvasively lifting and tightening skin over time." Their approach is to bypass the skin's surface and, through ultrasound heat, penetrate and stimulate deeper structural support layers of the skin, often in the same areas that surgery targets. This, in turn, is intended to create more collagen, which will build up over time, notably in two or three months, and sometimes generate continued improvements over an even longer period. The thirty- to sixty-minute in-office procedure is designed to do the trick...but can be a bit painful at first, according to lots of reviews available on the Web, which give the procedure generally good marks overall.

The results last more than a year, possibly two, when some go in for additional "firming." Physicians offering this FDA-approved procedure are increasingly widely available.

Science at work.

A stem-cell facelift, for another example, is a procedure gaining proponents, though without evidence-based research yet to back up claims or any standardized procedure. It is simply adding stem cells with their "potential" rejuvenating properties to a solution of body fat and then injecting it in the wrinkles and hollows in the face. Nonsurgical for sure—not proven as well. Yet one in what will no doubt be a long line of new procedures and techniques based upon anti-aging dreams and science.

DID YOU SAY "FACELIFT"?

Sorry to be a bit of a tease, but this book isn't about actual facelifts—or about not having them. It is about facelifts in the sense of aging with attitude and the decisions one makes through the decades. It is about "facelift" as a catchall term for dramatic, invasive attempts by women (and men) to suddenly turn back time or significantly alter nature.

UNDER THE KNIFE (OR NEEDLE)
ACROSS THE GLOBE

America leads the world by far in cosmetic surgery procedures each year. Second? China, and growing at an astonishing rate. Surprise, surprise. Third? Brazil. And France, a country devoted to female beauty and where women of a certain age are models of desire, elegance, and seductiveness? Not even in the top ten. French women seek a more natural look and feel, opting for creams and scrubs. Before considering the operating room, they focus on how they dress and groom and what they eat. And, as I've noted earlier, when they turn to the scalpel, it is for a little liposuction incision.

While the United States is well known for its nip-and-tuck-obsessed citizens, it actually does not have the greatest amount of plastic surgery *by percentage of population.* That title goes to South Korea. In fact, a 2009 study showed that 20 percent of South Koreans have had some sort of plastic surgery, a large majority identified as liposuction or double eyelid surgery, which helps create the illusion of more Western-looking eyes. In fact, this surgery is very popular across all of Asia.

Greece was second, with the majority of surgeries being breast augmentation. And though it's been known for ages to be the home of naturally beautiful women, Italy was number three, with a surprising amount of Botox procedures and liposuction.

It's no surprise that Brazil makes the list at number four, a country that has no stigma about plastic surgery—quite the contrary, it's often seen as a status symbol. In fact, the country has special government-based tax-deduction programs available for the hundreds of thousands of women who opt for breast implants. Number five on the list is Colombia, which has become a sort of destination for people from other countries to seek plastic surgery at a cheaper cost.

The United States ranks only sixth by population percentage, but it is estimated that Americans went under the knife or the needle more than 13 million times last year, far more than most of the countries above.

You can begin to see a correlation between the type of cosmetic surgery and how the nation values beauty. It's not surprising to see high rates of breast augmentation and liposuction in "Westernized" countries like the United States, Italy, and Greece, where the idealized woman is shapely but thin with large breasts—and usually scantily clad.

Then there is Asia. There is a stretch in Seoul, South Korea, with two hundred–plus plastic surgery clinics touting the latest and greatest in medical expertise and technology. The so-called "Beauty Belt" is a renowned destination in Asia and for Asians living elsewhere in the world. Unlike the West, where breast procedures, liposuction, and facelifts are popular, Asians often like to change their faces and bodies to look like their favorite celebrities. Really. Eyelid, nose, and facial bone surgeries are common. If you want a new chin, you might consider joining the 150,000 or so medical tourists who visit the Beauty Belt (the vast majority Chinese), but that would be about "beauty" and probably fantasy, and not about aging with attitude.

YES, I SAID "FACELIFT": OPTIONS

I have come to feel that it is a woman's right to decide for herself about facelifts. I don't have to agree. And there are clear-cut cases that demand plastic-surgery-cum-facelift, such as a disfiguring accident.

I have a friend in her sixties who was in the back of a New York City taxi that, while zooming along, lost its brakes. She found herself inside a restaurant, in the back of the taxi, bleeding profusely from wounds on her face where she hit the divider between the backseat and the front seat. In the ambulance she somehow had the presence of mind to call a friend to have her call her plastic surgeon to meet her at the hospital. She was going to need a real pro to minimize scarring and other adverse facial effects. And while it turned out her lacerations weren't all that bad (a lot of the blood came from a broken nose), she was going to be black-and-blue for weeks and sporting stitches. Being a New York opportunist, she not only ended up with a nose job and a facelift, and two months later looking more refreshed and healthy and years younger, she managed to get her medical insurance and the driver's accident insurance to pay for it.

Probably the first serious conversation I ever had about facelifts was in my fifties when a Southern belle who is an interior designer came to my home in Manhattan, on the recommendation of a neighbor, to help me understand a project. She was a stylish and attractive woman with bleached-blonde hair, a charming and chatty accent, and a way with words. Within five minutes of meeting her, she was chatting away about her next facelift like she was talking about going to the dentist. And did I want the name of her plastic surgeon? I literally was stunned. I had never encountered anything or anyone like this. Her behavior was so un-French. Not just talking about facelifts so openly and routinely, she was selling facelifts as if she got a big commission. While I managed to mumble a few questions, though I said it was a conversation, it was really a tour de force monologue. Amazing.

Why I remember it most is that I kept thinking, *If you are, say, fifty-five, and look pretty good for your age, why do you want another facelift? How are you going to look when you are seventy and working on your third or fourth facelift?* Ridiculous? Unnatural, certainly. There's no disguising the rest of one's body from one's face, such as wrinkled, spotted, or flabby hands and arms, though there are attempts to do so, and new technologies and treatments will surely be developed.

My takeaway point, then and now, is: really think hard about when is the right time, if any, to go under the scalpel. And certainly unless you are in a car accident or have some health reason, my advice is to wait. The number of women who have plastic surgery in their thirties and forties (breast enhancements and reductions excluded) is startling.

Regarding actual facelifts, the options are pretty simple, and the techniques are increasingly effective and targeted.

Broadly speaking, a facelift, in medical jargon a rhytid-ectomy, involves tightening the full facial muscles and skin, removing wrinkles, and lifting the face, with notable effect on the lower face, jowls, and neck. Subsets include:

- Browplasty: literally lifting someone's brow or fore-head and raising eyebrows.
- Blepharoplasty: the eyelid surgery that can reduce or reshape eyelids for aesthetic or medical reasons, remov-ing excess fat and skin on the upper eyelids and puffi-ness; sometimes includes the addition of permanent eyeliner.
- Otoplasty: ear surgery that can reshape the ears, though mostly just to pin protruding ears closer to the skull.

- Midfacelift: surgery that tightens the cheeks, which can also be augmented through implants, as can the chin.
- Lip enhancement.
- Necklift.

If you are contemplating getting a facelift, you obviously will want and need a lot more information. And here my advice is right out of my business background: get three bids. That is, after doing your online and word-of-mouth research, visit three surgeons for opinions before making a decision on what kind of surgery would be beneficial, when to have it, and by which physician.

To come full circle and return to the notion of a noninvasive, sustained beauty program, let me return to something of which I am sure about the French. As I mentioned, France is a country of creams and moisturizers and, let me add, facials. Probably both the products and the processes are one of its signature exports, though now those things have mostly lost any national identity. Still, the big cosmetics companies tend to be French, Japanese, or American. And a French name seems to connote top quality, even if the product is from another country.

When I grew up and went to college in Paris, the stores were a wonder of creams and treatments. They were part of my idea of a French woman. And even in my small town, Mother went for a facial twice a year. When I settled in Manhattan, people looked at me strangely when I asked where they went to get their facials. They didn't. I wound up going to a spa in Saks Fifth Avenue, where eastern European women took their work and professions very seriously. The cost was more than I could comfortably afford, but it was not a question of a luxury, it was just what a woman had to do to maintain a healthy skin. It was like going to the dentist for a cleaning—okay, not exactly—but it was considered required maintenance. Things are a little different today. You can even find rabbit on some menus in New York.

NATURE TO THE RESCUE: FOOD LIFTS

Face-friendly foods will help you put off the facelift question by giving your face a bit of a lift through nutrition. Certainly there are many things one can consider before contemplating the operating room, and cooking and eating well are much more enjoyable than recovering from plastic surgery! So have you eaten your spinach today?

Spinach is a great source of the antioxidant lutein, which helps prevent wrinkles by retaining the skin's moisture, which in turn also increases elasticity.

In general, diets rich in antioxidants and omega-3 fatty acids are face-friendly. Antioxidants are the enemies of the free radicals that help produce wrinkles, and increased lipids prevent dryness within our bodies and in cells from showing up on the outside.

You probably already know that oily fish and certain oils

are good for you, and that berries in particular are rich in antioxidants. Spinach and some other leafy green vegetables are also good sources of vitamins K and C, which may help reduce those dark circles under the eyes (unless those circles are a genetic trait or you have recently pulled too many all-nighters).

Oysters can help those dark circles, too, if they are related to iron or vitamin B_{12} deficiencies. Oysters are one of my favorite foods—I think I could eat them every day, though I have not tested that theory beyond perhaps four days. They are a miracle of nutrition, low in calories and loaded with wonders for the body (omega-3 fatty acids, vitamin E, magnesium, zinc, potassium, and high in protein). Plus, they come in all sorts of sizes and shapes and tastes.

I ate a lot of spinach and oysters growing up, and I continue to eat them wherever I am. I do not recall ever eating **avocados** in France, though, till relatively recently. I was introduced to them in New York and the Caribbean, but in today's global marketplace, they are everywhere. I love them, and I am delighted to know this newfound love has great anti-inflammatory properties, helping with skin blemishes and worse skin conditions. Oysters are a rich source of omega-3 fatty acids, which, as noted, provide moisture and flexibility to the skin, and increase collagen production to help us battle wrinkles. Not convinced? They also contain high levels of vitamin E, another warrior against aging.

Vitamin E is an exceptionally strong antioxidant and fights the evil free radicals. By our late thirties our bodies produce more free radicals than antioxidants. So a healthy supply of vitamin E helps delay wrinkles by protecting the collagen fibers in our skin against natural oxidation. One problem is that the body does not store vitamin E, so we need to ingest sufficient amounts as part of our diet. Avocados, spinach, and oysters all are good sources, as are nuts, vegetable oils, papayas, and eggs. Vitamin E also slows the growth of plaque in our arteries, thereby reducing the risks of atherosclerosis, and thus the risks of high blood pressure and heart disease. So eat your avocados, and your oysters, and your spinach.

Your skin will thank you if you also include some **bananas** in your diet. They, too, are face-friendly. The bananas in France always taste different to me than those in America, and of course they are smaller. Even bananas are supersized in my adopted homeland. The varieties imported into France generally come from Africa and Martinique, whereas those in North America are generally from Central and South America and the Caribbean. But all the bananas have the same health traits. They fight fluid retention and so can reduce puffiness around the eyes and face. Bananas are especially potassium rich (as are strawberries) and can neutralize high sodium content resulting from the intake of processed and fast foods or a heavy hand with the saltshaker. Fiber packed and a source of carbohydrates, bananas are also a natural combatant to high blood pressure and rich in vitamin B_6, which acts as an anti-inflammatory agent.

Here are some recipes to give you a jump start in incorporating these four face-friendly foods into your diet:

Spinach Salad with Mushrooms and Parmesan

Talk about balanced and healthy…spinach, mushrooms, Parmesan, and olive oil. This is one of my favorite brunch-lunch salads.

SERVES 4

4 tablespoons olive oil

7 ounces shiitake mushrooms, cleaned and sliced (cremini or white work fine, too)

1 tablespoon chopped fresh thyme

2 tablespoons sherry vinegar

Juice and zest of a lemon

10 ounces baby spinach, washed and dried

⅓ cup pine nuts, toasted

½ cup Parmesan shavings (use a vegetable peeler)

Salt and freshly ground pepper

1. Warm 1 tablespoon of the olive oil in a frying pan over medium heat. Sauté mushrooms until tender, about 8 minutes. Season to taste and add thyme. Remove pan from heat and cool to room temperature.

2. In a small bowl, mix the remaining 3 tablespoons olive oil with sherry vinegar and lemon juice and zest, and season to taste. Place spinach in a large bowl and add pine nuts and mushrooms. Pour vinaigrette over salad, toss to combine, and garnish with Parmesan shavings. Serve immediately.

Emulsion of Oysters on a Fondue of Spinach

For those who are not yet "into" raw oysters, this warm oyster recipe is bound to make you reconsider. It's my version of the famous oysters Rockefeller, which are yummy, but to my palate all those breadcrumbs and garlic detract from the oysters. I prefer the poaching method (much faster, too), and with a bit of butter create more of an emulsion (a more sensual word that fits with the "aphrodisiac" oyster). You can ask your fishmonger to shuck the oysters and keep the liquid and shells so you are all set to go.

SERVES 4

1 tablespoon olive oil
10 ounces baby spinach, washed and dried
¼ cup crème fraîche (sour cream works, too)
24 fresh oysters, shucked, liquor reserved (should have about ¼ cup oyster liquor)
2 tablespoons butter, chilled and cut into small pieces
Salt and freshly ground pepper

■　■　■　■

1. Warm the olive oil in a frying pan over medium heat. Add spinach, season with salt, and cover. Cook for 4 minutes, stirring occasionally with a wooden spoon. Uncover and continue cooking until spinach is wilted and tender, about 2 minutes. Drain any excess water from pan, stir in crème fraîche, and season to taste. Reserve in a warm place.

2. After filtering the oyster liquid, warm it in a saucepan over medium heat, skimming away foam. Add the oysters and cook until edges curl, about 1 minute. Remove from heat.

3. To serve, divide spinach among 4 small, shallow bowls. Remove oysters with a slotted spoon and place on top of spinach. Bring oyster liquor to a boil and whisk in chilled butter. Season to taste and pour over oysters and spinach. Serve immediately.

Note: For leek lovers, replace spinach with boiled leeks.

Avocado with Lemony Vinaigrette

For me, this wonderful fruit is best with a simple salad dressing. I eat avocados this way at least several times each month for lunch or as a side dish with a bigger meal. Among hundreds of recipes for using avocados, the most common preparation save au naturel is as guacamole, which I am not crazy about because of the usual tomato combo plus onions and/or garlic. Avocados and tomatoes are two of my favorite fruits, but when it comes to savoring them, I'd rather not have them together.

SERVES 4

2 ripe avocados

Coarse salt and freshly ground pepper

Juice of 1 lemon

1 teaspoon sherry vinegar

1 tablespoon olive oil

1 tablespoon chopped fresh basil (parsley and coriander are good alternatives)

1. Slice avocados in half and remove the pit. Place each half on a small plate. Season to taste.
2. Mix the lemon juice, vinegar, and olive oil and pour over the 4 halves. Garnish with basil and serve.

Banana, Orange, and Peanut Butter Croque Madame

I go bananas for bananas (forgive the pun), the perfectly pre-packaged fruit. I often eat half a banana with a knife and fork for dessert the French way, to avoid the all-too-common "gulping down" of food. It still is my favorite way, as a purist, of eating a banana, but then I am gourmande, too, and have enough banana recipes to fill a cookbook. I like them with cereal and yogurt, like most of us, but I also often make them flambé with a touch of rum for an elegant but easy dessert; banana cake ain't bad either. Banana pie is a treat I discovered as an exchange student in Weston, Massachusetts, and I love it. Banana smoothies can be dangerously delicious and fattening, but healthy, too, thanks to a banana's many nutrients.

A few years ago, a bunch of girlfriends were at the house in Provence (Americans and some Parisians who had lived and worked in New York) around Thanksgiving time when berry season is over. Somehow our fondness for peanut butter came up, and next we were playing around with the oh-so-French croque-monsieur, and we created an easy-but-filling lunch variation on the same theme. We had a bunch of bananas on the counter… the rest follows. Addiction guaranteed.

SERVES 2

4 slices sourdough bread (whole wheat or brioche works well, too)

2 tablespoons peanut butter

Zest of 1 orange

2 medium bananas, peeled and thinly sliced

1 tablespoon butter, softened

1 teaspoon sugar

Sprinkle of cacao powder (optional)

1. Place 2 slices of bread on a work surface and spread each with a thin layer of peanut butter. Sprinkle with orange zest and cover with a layer of banana slices. Top each with a second slice of bread. Lightly butter both sides and sprinkle with sugar.

2. Warm a large nonstick frying pan over medium heat. Add sandwiches and cook, pressing down lightly with a spatula, until golden brown (about 4 minutes per side).

3. Transfer the sandwiches to a cutting board, slice diagonally, add some cacao powder (if using), and serve immediately.

Note: To make a traditional-looking croque-monsieur, you may want to trim the bread crust and make 4 perfect squares.

4

THE ART AND MAGIC OF GROOMING

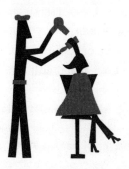

Alas, my wizard Parisian hairstylist of the past twenty-five years, Peter, just retired. He was one of my secret weapons in my attack on aging. He surely trimmed five years off me.

Peter was probably the world's slowest haircutter. Before he did anything, he concentrated...on one's hair, face, profile, the shape of one's head. He observed how you spoke, dressed, moved...any detail that would help him emphasize your style. In salon speak, this is called "the art of consultation" and the sign of a good stylist. Two people never got the same cut...and over time I never quite got the same cut. Sometimes the changes he made were subtle; sometimes the style shifted seemingly dramatically as I aged, but not in any wild or trendy way. I always felt my best leaving his salon.

Unlike anyone else who has cut my hair, Peter took one

hour just for cutting. He cut my hair three times. Each time, I would think he was finished, and he would get that look and stare and concentrate (he barely spoke), and then he began again. His cuts were so technically perfect they would last three or four months and still draw wows on the street. Not a great businessman, but a true and passionate artist.

Do you have a great hairstylist? If not, why not? Do you have a great haircut? If not, time to get one. Do you have a cut that helps define your brand and suits your age? If not… What does the mirror say?

Ah, but finding a great hairstylist? It always amuses me when I have a recent haircut and a stranger says to me, "Amazing haircut." And many people have said to me, "May I ask who cut your hair?" Flattery, sure, and when I say, "I had it cut in Paris," they say something like "I should have known," or "Of course." Asking someone with a cut you like, though, is one way to find a good hairstylist. Asking friends can help—and that is how I found Peter—but it doesn't always work out the first time, so be prepared for some trial and error. I remember having a cut in a city one day, and two days later having another one to fix the first one's mistakes.

I am always reminded that people notice your hair first, then your eyes and smile, and sooner, rather than later, your shoes. Somehow these are the areas we seem to focus on and use to make our first and often lasting assessment of a person's appearance and overall look. When you meet people you have not seen in a while and they say, "You look good," what are they using to make that call? All of the above, plus probably the tone of your complexion and the size of your waistline.

I know a woman in New York who is ninety and in the past couple of years has suffered from increasing dementia. Sad, of course. She was always very old-school about her appearance, dressing carefully with understated formality and style, and taking lots of care with her makeup, skin, and hair. Her entire adult life, she had a weekly appointment at the "beauty parlor," and still does. When you see her after one of her appointments, you look at her as if time stood still. Here is the woman you knew a decade ago.

I imagine her salon has plenty of experience in taking care of the hair of "older ladies." Perhaps there should be a branch of gerontology for hair maintenance . . . and certainly a chain of salons for women fifty-plus.

Let's face it, not only does one's hair get thinner with age—and one can lose a lot of hair—but one's face changes.

HOW TO DISCOVER THE BEST STYLE
FOR YOUR FACE

Mirror, mirror, what shape is my face? Oval, round, oblong, square, long, rectangular, triangular, inverted triangle, heart, diamond? Ah, but does that haircut you have chosen go with your face shape? And has your face shape changed with age? Gravity rules. As your skin becomes less elastic and your face droops (okay, falls), your oval face might become rounder or more square, especially if you have gained more than a soupçon of weight. Then what?

There are some obvious rules of thumb for hairstyles and

face shapes, such as: If your face is round, keep the sides trimmed around your ears and eyes. If your face is long, don't wear your hair long and straight, which will pull your face down even farther. But these basics are part of a bigger picture. Is your hair curly, wavy, or naturally straight? Are your hair strands thick, medium, or thin? Is your hair densely packed, or has it thinned so you can see your scalp? What color is your hair?

I wish I could give very specific advice and answers to you, but multiply ten facial shapes by forty common hairstyles and seemingly hundreds of not-so-common cuts, and there is enough to fill another book. It is worth the price to go to a top stylist at least once in a while, as he or she can advise you about the best cut for your face. And there are dozens of websites, articles, and books to consult. Things can get complicated if you let them. And keeping things simple, especially as one ages, is my mantra. A lot more goes into taking care of your hair than a virtual makeover (welcome the computer) or, if you are lucky, a blow-dry once or twice a week. The health of one's body and the grooming of one's hair are especially important (and related).

Your hair shows your attitude toward aging.

Mais, your hairstyle does not need to change with fashion and trends, so try to find one not too extreme that suits your face, personality, and lifestyle—one you can modify slightly over the years. Perhaps think of a hairstyle comparable to the timeless little black dress. Looking at classic icons of beauty such as Grace Kelly, Audrey Hepburn, Jacqueline Kennedy, or Catherine Deneuve, you'll notice that they changed their hairstyles only slightly throughout the years, though they played with the length a bit. After all, as with clothes, hair-styles come and go.

Your hair, like your skin, needs simple but consistent attention. Although genetics play a part, as we age we lose proteins in the hair strands and our hormones can wreak havoc at times, so it makes sense to take care of our mane.

I remember my *carré* or bob, à la Louise Brooks, starting when I was six, and here I am, decades later, still wearing a bob of sorts after many variations on the same theme (and a couple of years with long straight hair, *bien sûr*, during the usual fifteen-to-twenty-five age bracket): from parting in the middle to the side, with and without a bang, shorter or longer, a blunt cut or *plongeant* (that's short in the back, longer on the sides with layers on top in order to give it natural volume, and one that suits any type of hair), but still ze bob was what my long-time Parisian hairstylist said suited me best. Once in a while, when I felt like a change and showed him some pictures, Peter nixed the supershort or -long hair. Every time I resisted the change or the trim, it was not long before I became bored or didn't feel *bien dans ma peau* and went back to my familiar style. It's a classic hairstyle and as such never really falls out of style. True, the bob is about as timeless a cut as it gets today.

MAINTENANCE

You should plan a trim every two to three months to get rid of tired strands and keep your hair healthy. Many French women (*moi* included) believe that the right day to cut is on a full moon. Follow with a keratin-based structuring treatment for strong and supple hair. Fall is a good time to have a critical look at your hair to see if your hairstyle is still fresh and modern. The main idea is not to copy whatever is trendy, but to make sure the cut fits your personality and lifestyle of the moment. The goal is to have a style that suits your hair type so that you can do your hair easily (no chignon if your hair is superthin and sparse).

As adolescents we can certainly play with long hair, pigtails, and all the rest, but after forty, one should adopt a signature hairstyle, something simple but nothing so *coiffé* glamorous that it makes people turn around to look because it's ridiculously inappropriate (thus drawing attention to us and often to our age).

My friend Maguy and I saw just that extreme last spring while sitting outside the Palais Royal in Paris looking at passersby. A woman presumably in her seventies sat there with carrot-red hair (her white roots showing that she needed a retouch) and fake superlong eyelashes matching the hair color! As if this were not enough (maybe fashion week calls for the extreme), she had heavy blue eye shadow all over, and it was only early afternoon. Her clothes were normal and unremarkable, yet people looked at her more like they'd look at a clown or wondering if she had looked at herself in the mirror before stepping outside. We were trying to figure out her nationality, something harder and harder these days, but not a word came out of her, and we gave up, clueless. The point is: don't overdo it. Avoid extreme colors after your adolescence, though we saw plenty of pink- and blue-haired young girls that day who didn't shock or attract much notice from the crowd. The *poil de carotte* lady did, though not in a good way. Forget aggressive red-orange...or perhaps shiny blue-black for that matter. As we get older, we lose pigment in our skin. Deep, dark hair shades make wrinkles and pale skin stand out. Ditto for dark lipstick. A subtler shade of hair color is better for our complexions.

A SHAMPOO *PEUT-ÊTRE*?

Washing your hair daily is a very American concept, while the French are notorious for not washing their hair (or brushing their teeth) enough, although today both are a bit of a myth as hair rules have become international via global women's magazines and brands.

I know French women who wash their hair every other day and American women who do so twice a week. Ironically, plenty of US salons, which are not part of a chain or promoting a brand, use only French products; whereas the similar stylists in France love American products. Go figure. The eternal "We always want what we can't have" also seems to apply to hair stuff.

To the French defense, I'd say the reason we don't believe in washing our hair daily is that after our nightly skin-cleansing ritual we also have one for hair: put your head forward, and with a good-quality brush (a boar-bristle brush is the best investment), brush your hair in reverse to get rid of dust and give it some breathing. The only time we wash our hair daily is at the beach, where we use a mild shampoo with neutral pH (Kerium Doux Extrême from La Roche-Posay is a good one, and Garnier makes an effective range for different hair types).

No matter the type of hair, we still think a daily shampoo irritates the hair, accelerates the sebum secretion, and long term makes the hair weak and flat. Too much of a good thing ain't always wonderful. The way to shampoo is important, too: forget the extreme strong massage, which may force soapy chemicals into your scalp, but rather go for a quick, delicate caressing while gently massaging the roots with the pulp of your fingers. (A stimulating massage comes after you have rinsed out the soap and chemicals.) During the course of the year, two to three shampoos a week is plenty, a French-American compromise of sorts. And time-saving...

One needs to find the shampoo that's good for one's hair, and that can take a bit of doing. A treatment shampoo is always a good choice, but most important, no matter if your hair is dry or oily, is to pick two shampoos and alternate, as you don't want your hair to get used to the same active ingredients. That's somewhat difficult if you go to a salon, as they tend to use their brand or the one they affiliate with, so don't be shy about taking your own. Unlike the skin, hair fibers do not renew themselves every month (each hair normally lives four or five years), so it's always the same cells that absorb the active ingredients. Add a third type of shampoo once a month (the analogy is a mild detox), a clarifying shampoo that will eliminate the residue of hair products you've used as well as chlorine, pollution, and anything that makes your hair look dull. A product that will make your hair look shiny and healthy from Fekkai is their clarifying apple cider shampoo.

A shampoo always ends with a rinse, of course. The simplest, whether you have applied a conditioner or not—and don't limit to the summer—is to rinse your hair with a final cold dousing to help give it some further life and shine. (While I probably should have some scientific proof of that—I know it closes the pores and hair follicles—I trust a lifetime of advice and experience here regarding the life and shine.) Another nice rinse after each shampoo that reportedly helps limit hair loss is a mix of two tablespoons of cider vinegar with two tablespoons of honey in a quart or liter of water. Just rinse and leave it to do its magic. I also like to end with a rinse of lemon juice or red wine vinegar for maximum shine a couple of times a month. Again, alternate so as not to bore your hair!

With each shampoo, a final massage after the soap and chemicals have been initially rinsed out helps activate the roots. Start from the back of the neck and go over the sides of the ears and crown of the head; and if possible, wash your hair with your head down. All of this will activate the circulation and stimulate the follicles.

Another bit of extra tender-loving care is a weekly mask on one's hair. A good and quick one is the hydrating mask EverPure from L'Oréal, but you can also make some at home. My favorite is a teaspoon of olive or argan oil, and another good one is a mixture of avocado with olive oil and a few drops of lemon. Leave on your hair for twenty minutes after covering loosely with a plastic wrap (or shower cap).

BRUSHING

If brushings were bad for hair, most of us would have no hair left. Brushing is good, as I illustrated earlier.

My mother was vain about her hair and followed a not-uncommon old-world tradition. She never left her bedroom without her hair being perfect (or at least her interpretation of perfect). Plus, she never went to bed without brushing her hair.

My mother, who started to become gray in her forties, had her hair dyed light auburn into her eighties. More telling, though, was that no one really appreciated that she always had long hair. No one, save me on rare occasions, saw her long hair reaching to her waist. That's because she kept it pinned up all those years on the back of her head in a Simone de Beauvoir chignon (the name comes from *chignon du cou*, French for "nape of the neck"). When Mother retired for the evening, she took her hair down and brushed it in her bedroom. In the morning, she put it up again. My husband or anyone else who at times shared her home or traveled with her never saw her hair over her shoulders.

The key to a good blow-dry depends on who does it and how. Many young salon assistants nowadays do the blow-dry (I loved the days when your hairstylist did everything and got to understand your hair from shampoo to finish. A few in my world still do it, but they are the exception, not the rule), and assistants are often not properly trained and/or in a hurry and tend to overshampoo and use maximal heat (now that's heavy damage) on your hair. If this is not bad enough, they stick the dryer to your scalp, which irritates the hair and dries it out. It's okay if you go for a blow-dry occasionally, but on a regular basis you need to control damage. At home, it's always best to use medium heat, or better, wrap your hair in a towel for five to ten minutes of some natural drying, then brush the front and use your fingers to help shape your hair. An ionic blow-dryer is worth the investment if you do it yourself. The BaByliss Pro 2800 Super Turbo is a good value. You may want to use a few Velcro rollers (they are great for travel and have saved many bad hair days during my corporate life) if you are looking for a bit of body or a lift at the roots. If you use a good serum (another good occasional treat for your mane), you may be amazed to learn how little you need to do to look great without a fancy and time-consuming brushing and blow-dry. Going natural is also a good thing as we get older.

TO GO GRAY OR NOT TO GO GRAY;
THAT IS THE QUESTION

"There's a reason why forty, fifty, and sixty don't look the way they used to, and it's not because of feminism, or better living through exercise," notes Nora Ephron. "It's because of hair dye. In the 1950s only 7 percent of American women dyed their hair; today there are parts of Manhattan and Los Angeles where there are no gray-haired women at all."

I confess I am my mother's daughter, and I have yet to let myself go au naturel, whatever that may mean for me today.

Since I worked in a competitive world engaging only energetic, dynamic, and well-groomed women, I have had my hair colored since my fifties. Thanks to Peter, I have lightened it a shade or two and occasionally added highlights (the summer sun in Provence does both naturally). The lighter hair color makes me look and feel younger. I am sensitive, though, to the fact that if my complexion and hair color start to match, I look washed out. That is something to be sensitive to when choosing both hair color and makeup. I have a challenge in the summer, when my hair gets lighter and my skin darker, even while I watch my midday sun exposure and wear hats and creams all the time. Provence will be Provence. (A colored Panama hat is my secret weapon. I wear it; the hat changes color.) And as my godmother used to say about a hat: "Ça cache la misère" (It hides the miseries; read bad hair days).

So, coloring or no coloring? This is a major point of discussion for my friends in their early forties when the first gray hair appears and the panic starts. The first reaction, more often than not, is "I don't want to dye my hair." So, perhaps try a semipermanent hair color first. And there is always the option of trying a new haircut that satisfies for now and puts off the question a bit longer. For a less-than-drastic step, try henna. What most of us don't know is that once you've done color, henna is out forever. (Supposedly it reacts with the color set of some hair dyes.) Having been to Morocco first when I was in grad school, I envied the beautiful manes of Moroccan women (that's when I first learned about argan oil and henna) and witnessed a few of those natural treatments. They got it right.

For most of us the day comes when too many gray hairs neither look nor feel right, so the option becomes an obligation unless one chooses to let the gray grow until an all-over and uniform color that you can live with has been achieved. Some women, of course, look stunning with silver-gray hair. There's a signature item! Think Helen Mirren or Jamie Lee Curtis. For many of us, however, it's not an option if we have a career and want to look the part. Or because we have too fair a complexion, which is not happy with gray hair, or simply because we feel older with gray hair.

Covering gray hair is not the only reason to color one's hair. Many women find that a good color can take years off, especially with highlights. The key is subtlety so the hair looks brighter and not necessarily lighter.

Color: Do it at home or at the salon? That's a tough choice, as the salon is both expensive and time-consuming, but the home deal is risky! I know a few women who do their color at home and some got the hang of it, but usually it seems hit or miss. For me, knowing my ineptitude with blow-drying, I decided that it would be my luxury as well as my hour of relaxation to give the chore to someone who can do it better. I got lucky to last without coloring till my fifties, much older than my mother, who was gray at forty; but admittedly it's no fun once you are committed, as it's a repeat every five to six weeks (I refuse to do it once a month, which is the norm, so I cheat with the convenient little color stick found in the hair section of beauty products stores). It's not ideal or perfect, but it is easy, convenient, and saves a couple of weeks, and frankly I do it more to save on hair damage, even if we are told that color does not affect the hair...it does. Think about it: the stuff in hair color needs some good R & D, as we should have some without ammonia, and the first "organic" ones are still outrageously expensive and not foolproof.

Try to find someone local who is going to "know" your hair, someone you can trust, and then stay with him/her. It takes a while for someone to get a feel for your hair, and having experienced colorings in other cities and countries, I must say it's usually not the best. France has been an exception simply because the training, at least up to a few years ago, for a colorist or hairstylist is more rigorous than in most places. Or am I just being a Francophile? I have not seen too many of my friends, young or old, cry when they leave a French salon because the cut or the color or both are disasters. In New York, it's another story: even friends who go to the most expensive (French) salons have had too many bad experiences. If you come out with great cut and color...drop your anchor.

Summer is not so good for the hair, and it's especially bad for colored hair, especially if you spend time at the beach, in a pool or the sea. The sun and water can turn hair blonde, brassy, or worse, even greenish. (In the case of green—really more common than I would have imagined—the best trick is to put two aspirins in a bowl, pour a few drops of water on them to effervesce, add your shampoo, and mix into a paste. Apply to wet hair, leave on a few minutes, and shampoo as usual.) A lightweight shampoo without sulfites, like L'Oréal EverPure or Bumble and Bumble support conditioner, helps. Avoid immersing your hair underwater, and if you are outdoors between 11 a.m. and 4 p.m., wear a hat. The worst color for the sun damage, dark blonde (that's me), requires good care or it fades into dull streaks.

If you need to lighten your color for the summer, the old-school French way is to use olive oil as a cataplasm on your hair. The thick and heavy oil will dissolve the hair's excess color and patina.

A LITTLE MORE PROTECTION

Summer, of course, is a good time to avoid blow-drying and just air-dry your hair with your fingers and avoid potential damage to the already fragile follicles.

If you go for biking (like me) or hiking (not like me) out in the wind, it is better to wear your hair back and covered with a scarf. The key is to protect the hair from the sun: the rule is don't go out without a hat. Hats are back, in case you did not notice. After the summer, avoid *balayage* (highlights), and tone the color down one shade (or talk with a colorist about blending lowlights with the highlights).

One last thing regarding color is to avoid doing it right before a big event, as the color needs to set, and the day you do the color your hair is in a state of shock (at least that's how I see it), and even a great blow-dry is different from the usual. So schedule it a week before you want to look your best.

At menopause the hair can get an extra beating. Many women complain about the hair thinning and looking tired and dull or basically weak (it needs moisture big-time, like a plant). Have a blood test so your doctor can determine if you have enough of all the basic vitamins. Your immune system may also be running low, and the decrease in estrogen adds to the complications. Good nutrition is vital in the early fifties and will set you in shape for the next stages.

Feed your hair. Oysters are the food par excellence for strong, healthy hair at any age. Salmon, mackerel, sardines, nuts, green vegetables, carrots, and fresh fruits are also high on the list. Avoid processed foods, caffeine (watch the soda), junk food, and any food with lots of flour and sugar, like cupcakes and other cakes. They aren't great for your body, your mind, or your hair!

Losing a lot of hair can happen through life and to all of us. End of summer is the worst time for it, but then again it's natural and short term. Vichy, Dercos, and some other brands make stimulating cocktails with minerals that will help, and it's also good to use a lotion that revitalizes the hair during the night. Insufficiencies in iron, zinc, or proteins are usually to be blamed. So, ladies, eat your oysters.

Thin hair is most likely the worst, both for the customer and for the stylist. The magic solution is to get a scissor cut on dry hair to give it lightness and volume, a great technique. Thin hair is usually dry as well and needs to be hydrated (moisturize, moisturize, moisturize), but as it gets greasy and heavy with certain products, it's good to concentrate on hydrating waters like Bumble and Bumble Thickening or Schwarzkopf Professional Shampoo, which contain lactic acid and keratin and can protect the damaged scales. Always apply the shampoo into your hands first and gently work it into the hair, using the lather to wash your scalp. A conditioning is vital. A cream rinse can also help. Thin hair loves the sensual gesture of your fingers to dry it gently. Your additional magic solution is to opt for a cure of trace elements, amino acids, or vitamins.

Unusually damaged (often a lack of vitamin E) or dry (often a lack of vitamin A) hair requires some masks. Fekkai's shea butter is a good one to give back suppleness and elasticity to the hair. Make sure to take the time after you apply a mask to cover your hair with a warm towel and wait twenty minutes so the active ingredients penetrate well. Products with keratin are equally helpful, and so are hot oil treatments.

Dull hair (it's dull because it can't reflect the light) can benefit from oils before a shampoo. Aveda and Phyto make good ones; the latter has a wonderful Alès oil. Put on hair *raie par raie* (part by part), add to the ends, and leave on for twenty minutes before rubbing gently with warm water, and then do your normal shampoo.

Rebellious hair results when we are stressed or tired over a period of time, and the after-brushing serums are key to putting some luster back in the fiber and giving it a shiny coat. Look for products with silicon, such as Schwarzkopf's Göt2b Glossy Anti-Frizz Shine Serum, which works well as it coats each strand so the cuticle stays smooth. Distribute the serum with a wide-tooth comb (instead of a brush) and style with your hands. My friend Claudine deals with frizzy hair using John Frieda products, which will also add some shine. For weak hair, an additional deep-conditioning mask once a week is worth experimenting with. For any of us, a few drops of olive oil on dry ends always work...a little moisture in your mane is a good thing.

I have implicitly been writing about hair products and procedures that have a foundation in science, albeit often proven by experience and not impartial scientific studies. But as with anti-aging skin care and variations on facelifts, science will certainly bring the post-forty generation of baby boomers many new products to counter what is fact. Yes, our hair gets thinner; we lose perhaps 30 percent of our follicles; hair texture changes with age and hormonal shifts; and our hair becomes more fragile from exposure to all the chemicals we are putting on it and from the sun's UV rays. However, savvy scientists and cosmetics companies are at work this very instant to address each condition. Expect a bag of individual hair treatments in your not-too-distant future. Again, science and commerce at work.

Each hair texture has its charm, temperament, and exigencies. Like your skin, it requires you to get to know it and work with it in order to embellish it. Good nutrition and health will resolve 80 percent of your hair challenges, and good care will do the rest.

5

BEAUTY AND SOME MAKEUP AND MANICURES

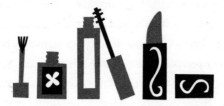

We use moisturizers, wear makeup, trim our toenails, and wear smexy (smart and sexy) clothes and shoes to approach feeling or looking beautiful. But beauty in whose eyes? Standards for beauty have been different through the ages and cultures and continue to evolve. (Or there would no longer be fashion designers and the like.) Right now, the world seems fixated on a global standard of an American-and-Western-inspired look: a youthful homogenized look that is heavily promoted. Add slim bodies but big breasts and an uptilted narrow nose. Remember all the Asians who get plastic surgery to look like someone else? And consider this: Iran has begun to see soaring rates of rhinoplasty, the nose being one of the very few physical aspects that is seen on the usually burka-clad women of the country who claim that a softer,

"Western" nose is more beautiful. The surgery is so popular there that Tehran has been dubbed the "Nose Job Capital" of the world.

Also add tall, as in tall models, to the abnormal image of beauty being touted today in a Western fashion-designer way. What are all those platform shoes and five-inch heels really about? Watch an award show like the Oscars broadcast globally and you will see beautiful actresses, dressing like models. After fasting painfully (and complaining about it publicly to bond with their audience), these actresses are squeezed into gowns (often with skin fully exposed on their backs and sometimes shoulders) that are loaned by a famous fashion house and designer. Their hair is elaborately styled and frozen in place, and their makeup is camera perfect. Then they are jacked up four or five inches to appear abnormally tall. And that is our ideal of beauty today? It certainly would not pass Renoir's test.

I am struck by this evolution toward "extreme beauty." This kind of look certainly cannot fit all. So I wonder about all those designer gown knockoffs. Who wears them? Young fashionista wannabes at weddings? Certainly not women who age with attitude. Plus, I always think it a little foolish to rush to the flavor-of-the-season look. It is something that's forgiven in the young perhaps, but not for the rest of us. And again, notions of beauty are fickle.

Consider beauty as it was promoted in the West in the 1920s in magazines and movies.

In 1920, a very pale complexion with blushed cheeks was a popular makeup look, paired with bright, bloodred lipstick. But the moment the inimitable Coco Chanel appeared in public with the faint signs of a suntan, our love affair with a more sun-kissed look got started.

By 1929, with pale out and tan in and considered healthy, cosmetics company Coty helped women achieve the increasingly popular sunless tan. Coty Tan self-tanning powder and liquid was formulated to "beat the sun at its own game." Many decades later, the cosmetics industry of today continues to "perfect" tan in a bottle or jar. And along came technology and tanning salons across nations, as unhealthy as some may be. But I get it; I hide from the damaging rays of the sun and wear sunscreen routinely, yet I am culturally conditioned to feel better when I have my August hue. Perhaps someday we will return to "new-and-improved" painted faces of the court of France during Louis XIV's reign as again the *ne plus ultra* of beauty. Painted beauty marks are something to contemplate as we age.

FIVE OR SIX WISE WORDS ON MAKEUP

Skin care and makeup are, of course, not the same thing, though they increasingly overlap for the good. A touch of lipstick, for example, is an essential lip moisturizer. But what color lipstick? Is fire-engine red still the right one at age fifty, sixty, seventy, eighty? (It was in the 1930s when sales of red lipstick soared, with oxblood being one of the most popular shades of the time. Amusingly, its downside was that it often stained your lips and the lips of anyone you happened to kiss while wearing it!)

Here are two realities: (1) bad makeup, as in boldly penciled-in eyebrows, too much eyeliner on the upper and lower lids, coloring-book colors, et cetera, et cetera, makes one look like a clown at best and grotesque at worst; and (2) too much makeup, especially as one ages, generally makes one look worse rather than better.

Makeup in the hands of an artist, of course, can do wonders. The right touch of makeup is a style accent and rejuvenator par excellence. But here's an irony: When you are young, you don't need much makeup, but you can wear it well. When you are old, you think and you may indeed need more cover-ups and accents, but you cannot wear them well.

A problem we all face with getting makeup advice is that the people who give it are in the business of either selling makeup products or applying makeup products. How do we learn what is best for us as we age?

I don't have a really good answer beyond trial and error and looking hard and objectively in the mirror.

But, as noted, I do have a mantra: "Less is more."

A touch of lipstick, sure. A thin line of eyeliner, sure. A little cover-up base and a little worked-in color to raise one's cheeks and eyes, sure. Then you are on your own. Most of the time, you want to look yourself, which means consistency. And makeup, unlike hair coloring, really cannot turn back the clock dramatically, but can just make you look your best for your age. Contrariwise, bad makeup à la heavy foundation and mascara can make you look your age—deepening wrinkles and making your eyes look older—and more. Light and well-done makeup, on the other hand, can make you look more rested, more polished, and help you feel more attractive and confident.

Let me cover a few more specific approaches and details to makeup that help us address nature's realities in a cosmetic but not medical fashion.

First, the base. For most of us, after forty, foundation and other coverage base makeup such as concealer and powder are our most frequently used beauty staples and friends—but if they're not used correctly, they can easily become foes. Personally, I am a minimalist.

It may seem counterintuitive, but as we age we need *less* makeup, not more. "Less is more" is a tenant I preach for many things, and when it comes to makeup and aging, not practicing it is a serious mistake. The more fine lines and wrinkles you have, the more sparingly you need to apply your foundation and especially your powdered base. Too much and the makeup actually begins to seep into and accentuate the lines on your face, not conceal them. And another tip, by the way: once your face has noticeable wrinkles, don't even think about makeup and moisturizers with glittery particles that draw attention. *C'est tout.*

Instead of piling it on, choose a sheer or lightweight liquid foundation or a tinted and luminescent moisturizer. These brighten the skin and give the impression that the skin is glowing. And who doesn't want to glow? Dior Airflash is an aerated foundation, which is great for minimal makeup users. It gives the skin that airbrushed look. (It's best to pull hair up in a towel and apply without a blouse on so you don't get spray on your hair or clothes.)

If you ever have your makeup done professionally or have seen it done on TV, you'll notice the artists rarely use their fingers to apply base makeup, and instead opt for a foundation brush or a soft sponge. These tools help distribute the makeup evenly and sparingly. They're also much gentler and do not stretch the skin as our fingers can. To apply, dot the foundation in small circles on your problem areas only and then softly use the brush to work into the skin.

Apply a bit of powder on the nose, forehead, and chin to reduce shininess if needed, but use sparingly. Too much powder makes the skin look dry and accentuates fine lines. This is why most makeup artists abide by a golden rule, especially when working with women over forty: no powder around the eyes.

And speaking of eyes, it's important to note: the skin under our eyes begins to thin as we get older. Take special care not to stretch or pull on this delicate area. Most women begin to see fine lines, crow's-feet, and dark circles around their eyes after forty—and inevitably reach for the thick concealer stick to mask these issues. However, too much can actually accentuate what they're trying to cover up. Instead, use a lightweight liquid concealer or foundation and apply sparingly with a brush, avoiding the inner eye area. Maybelline roll-on eraser/concealer for eyes is very affordable, effective, and easy to apply. Makeup guru Bobbi Brown, though, favors a light concealer there to make you look less tired—and her creamy concealer is a flawless, quality product. Better yet is more sleep and being less tired!

Depending on your tastes, you can apply eye shadow, eyeliner, mascara, or all three. I tend to keep it simple in this area. A bit of eye shadow in a neutral color with some reflective particles helps to brighten the eyes but not overpower them. A little eyeliner that's very thin (or almost nonexistent) toward the inner part of the eye and thicker toward the outer part of the eye helps to counterbalance the natural and inevitable little droop that happens as our time goes on. And when eyeliners no longer achieve the effect you want, use, for example, the appropriately named matte color Faux Pas from Lancôme, which takes three seconds to smear and results in both an eyeliner and a bit of shadow.

In America, and it seems to me in what I've seen of the Middle East, for a special occasion a smoky eye has become a classic—no idea why. But no matter your age, it's best suited for an evening event such as a wedding or gala. Even then, keep it simple and subtle. But frankly, I just don't get putting on a face for a special occasion that isn't your own...never have.

One "rule" to always abide by is to steer clear of the bottom of the eye. Eyeliner and mascara on the lower lashes actually make the eyes look smaller. After a few hours, it also begins to creep down and settle into the fine lines around the eyes, accentuating dark circles—exactly what you *don't* want. At least I don't.

To add a little pop of color? We all feel more beautiful when we have some color in our cheeks. It's a term that extends far beyond vanity, serving as an indicator for health and vitality. However, rosy cheeks are best reserved for cherubs and children. As we age, applying blush to the apples of the cheeks can actually draw attention to sagging skin. *Quelle horreur!* Instead, use a large blush brush and apply starting at the highest part of your cheekbone, usually just below your eye, and sweep away from the center of your face, upward toward the space between your eye and ear. No matter your skin tone, stay away from deep shades and blushes that have a brown or copper base to them (such as bronzers). They can actually make the skin look sallow. Instead, opt for a rose or a peach base, which will brighten and illuminate the skin. Also, many experts suggest a cream blush versus a powder blush for older women.

The lips: *ooh la la.* It's been said—and even studied— that men find lips to be the most sensual part of a woman. So it's no wonder so many women spend years adorning their lips with colors and glosses that emphasize them, making the wearer feel sexier and more noticed, too.

Alas, as we age, the skin isn't the only part of the face that sees the effects of time. The lips begin to fade in color and thin out (hence why many women of a certain age turn to collagen injections). They also begin to form very small fine lines (similar to what happens around our eyes). *C'est la vie.* But what many women don't realize is that when it comes to lips, as we age, the "Less is more" maxim applies as well.

So it's out with the "bold." Bright neon colors and deep, dark shades are too heavy for thinning lips. This is one case where I don't recommend a good merlot. Instead, pick a neutral rose shade, which looks good on most skin tones. Also consider a sheer gloss—it will give you more fullness without overpowering the lips.

In the end, consistency is important, as is being comfortable in your own skin. I learned some lessons the hard way, and I have the photos and videotapes to prove it. I am not a fan of extreme makeovers. Or anything more than a tweaking of what comes naturally to you. In my professional life, I had to use makeup artists for television appearances so many times I am almost embarrassed to say. They did not succeed in making me into Catherine Deneuve. Sometimes they succeeded in making me not me. There once was a time, for instance, when all the major morning TV shows had serious makeup artists for the guests. Sitting for one was an obligatory part of appearing on the show. I never found two the same, nor did I look the same, including when I had back-to-back appearances on two networks. I always got talked into a little of this and a little of that. Perhaps one in five or maybe ten made me look my best, and that only encouraged me to give the next person a try. Stupid me. Now the anchors have people who know their skin, their face, their needs, the setting, and even the products that work best for them. These are the real artists, and they work with the same customers repeatedly to find what is best for them. Of course, camera lights require a type of makeup you would not wear on the street.

My moment of committing to "Less is more" occurred at the Academy Awards. This falls under the category of "it is hard work but someone has to do it"! In my champagne days working for LVMH and Veuve Clicquot, I used to go to Hollywood for the awards and parties (I am smiling). If you are booked at any one of a half dozen hotels where the "stars" and industry moguls are staying, you are swept up with goody bags and free this and that, even offers to borrow designer gowns and clothes if you are going to be in the spotlight—and you want to dress and look good. It is *the* night—practically the only night—Hollywood dresses up, and everyone wants to look amazing. I used to accept a free blow-dry and makeup session at a salon on Rodeo Drive. (By the way, "free" in those days meant you left a hundred-dollar tip on what would have been a hundred-dollar salon bill, even though it would have been a twenty-five-dollar tab in most neighborhood places.) I know why I got the blow-dry. The makeup...well, I was there. I went to the salon looking like myself. I looked better after the blow-dry, but after the makeup? I walked out looking fine, but just not like me. I knew I was going to a costume party, but I preferred my own face.

NAILS, NAILS, AND AGE

Nail treatment can be categorized as another form of makeup, tellingly so, but like hair, nails age and demand different treatments over time. Certainly nails, like hair, can make a powerful grooming statement. Remember the woman with carrot-colored hair at the Palais Royal? Just a suggestion, but after the age of forty, don't consider carrot-colored or bright, boldly colored nails. Okay? More than color, well-manicured nails are about being well-groomed and, sure, pampering oneself a bit. It's a good thing, a positive, and a mood enhancer.

Nails grow slower as you age and often become more

brittle and dull. Unhealthy nails, like unhealthy hair, can signal some deeper health problems, especially nutritional deficiencies (beware the effect of yo-yo diets on your nails, especially those laden with protein). In advancing years, nails may become yellowed and opaque and may develop ridges. All this is natural, as is greater thickness and hardness, particularly of one's toenails. Just the invitation for some polish or buffing as a normal part of grooming and attitude as one ages.

It seems to me that painting one's nails was once an at-home activity or perhaps an occasional hair salon *supplément*. That has all changed over the past decade in New York and beyond. Nail salons have proliferated like coffee bars. Fact: within one thousand yards or meters of my Manhattan home, there are at least seven nail salons. And as far as I can tell, they are reasonably busy...all of them. Having one's nails done has gone from being thought of as an inexpensive indulgence to a routine activity. (There are at least five coffee shops in the same small area!)

With so many people going to nail salons for manicures and pedicures, often for procedures that one cannot manage by oneself at home, the push for more, not less, is evident. These nail technicians constantly upsell their processes and procedures to enhance their bills and tips. That is the way of the world. But it does not mean it is wise to add sparkles to your artificial purple nails. By the way, while the latest acrylic manicures are relatively safe—though they can thin and/or crack the nail plate—they can cause allergic dermatitis, and after removal, fungal and bacterial infections are all too common.

Remember, less is more as one ages, and nail care needs to coordinate with hair care and makeup. One of the telltale signs of age that cosmetic surgery has yet to conquer is the back of one's hands. Do you want to draw attention to yours with bright or flashy nail polish or superlong nails? Enough said.

I welcome the little luxury of a manicure and pedicure done by trained others, especially as competition has kept the prices down. I can even get a manicure or pedicure at most airports, though I don't. However, I recently encountered the logical extension into absurdity: a fish pedicure. In Saint-Rémy-de-Provence, an entrepreneur is cashing in on tourists sitting in chairs with their feet submerged in a boxlike tank, where tiny fish nibble at the dead cuticles around their toenails. It is reported not to work as well as scissors and cuticle removers. Should I ever try, I will be sure to get an appointment early in the day when the fish are still hungry.

6

ONCE A DAY, A LITTLE INVISIBLE EXERCISE

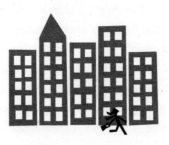

What happens to aging dancers? If you are a professional ballroom dancer, probably you waltz into the sunset. But a professional ballet dancer, like most professional athletes, has a limited career in her prime, and often an injury ends that career, sometimes prematurely. Then what? Teaching? Or something completely new and different? Fortuitously, I have found them in the emerging *bien-être* (health and wellness) business. These superb, well-trained and -educated athletes know the human body well, know training well, and stand out as yoga or exercise or Pilates or gyrokinesis teachers. They coach breathing and movement and even massage at an unusually high level in a field where too many relative amateurs with modest credentials tell you what to do with your body.

As part of my longtime lifestyle approach to taking care of my nothing-special body (it has always needed help), I've needed a little external coaching either to learn the right type of exercise or for imposed discipline (read overcoming inertia). I've required the mental push of a scheduled session, and from time to time I have needed help climbing the knowledge ladder. Living in New York, I have been fortunate to meet some of the finest teachers and coaches anywhere. Alicia is one of them.

Alicia is an ex-dancer from the New York City Ballet who, after a dozen years on the professional stage and at only age thirty, succumbed to injury (and a heart broken by a long-term lover) and transitioned to a career as a certified teacher in a number of the *bien-être* areas I mentioned. She is truly committed and gifted. Born in northern Europe, she decided a year ago she needed a change and moved to Paris, though she did not speak French.

I reconnected with her in Paris and found she is teaching in a center for Pilates. She loves Paris, is very happy, and has started to study French. "But how can you teach in Paris when you don't speak French?" I asked. "Easy," she said. "Most of my clients are expats or hotel guests and tourists."

Et voilà. Most of the French women I know, no matter their age, don't like the idea of "exercising" or "doing sports" in a room. It's cultural. Let's face it, for too many it's also a question of time (we'd rather do something else?), laziness, being a non-priority, requiring too much effort...and French women are notorious for avoiding anything that requires too much effort for too little pleasure.

How about you?

And yet...exercise slows the aging process. Proven. That's why I believe in incorporating movement (i.e., exercise, but I avoid that word because if physical activity is part of your lifestyle, it is not exercise) into my routine activities, like taking the stairs for a couple of floors rather than the elevator.

Conscious and habitual movement is a must for aging well, whether it is walking, taking the stairs, practicing yoga, dancing, swimming, biking, having sex—and, well, formal "exercising," especially post-sixty-five—or whatever it takes to move your *derrière* with joy (but please don't sweat and stress like so many celebrities who torture themselves a third of each day to stay fit. They'll die, too, no matter the intensity). Gravity spares no one.

Slow and easy wins the race (remember the tortoise, a French woman, and the hare?)—from walking to swimming to gyrokinesis. Shape your body. Breathe better. Sharpen your senses.

I love the recent French TV and movie theater campaign message with one little line: "Manger...bouger" (Eat and move your butt). The French are succumbing to globalization, and many are getting *un peu* rotund and some *trop*. Too bad the message is so often shown below junk-food advertising (and no bureaucrat sees that the government is wasting money as one is mesmerized by the junk above?). These two verbs, *eat* and *move*, go well together, and if done consistently (yes, moderation in both cases), you are bound to hit your last decades in good or even great shape. And you will also be happier: How is that for an added bonus? Tax-free!

SCIENCE (OR NATURE) SAYS

Let's not belabor the physical realities of growing old. If you have a little difficulty moving when you get out of bed and get going in the morning, you know what I am talking about...and if you don't, you will. But let's be realistic and recognize some of the physiological symptoms of aging and thus the advantages of an appropriate lifestyle incorporating physical activity.

We can understand wear and tear, especially in our joints and notably in our spines. Our connective tissues become less elastic, our lubricating fluids decrease, and our muscle fibers shorten. We slow down, *enfin*. Provence is just the place to experience this. The local motto is "Doucement le matin, pas trop vite l'après-midi, lentement le soir" (Gently in the morning, not so fast in the afternoon, and slowly in the evening).

We lose muscle mass through the decades (it starts in our twenties, alas), and with that, strength and endurance. It is not uncommon to be down 30 to 40 percent in muscle mass by age seventy. And since motor neurons die, particularly after age sixty, and we also lose more fast-twitch muscle fibers than slow-twitch, we lose quickness as well as balance.

Starting as early as twenty-five, our cardiovascular systems begin to decline. Our heart rates decrease by five to ten beats a minute per decade. Our oxygen-intake capacity decreases about 5 percent per decade. Big oxygen-carrying blood vessels stiffen, and blood pressure rises. Our respiratory systems can decline 40 to 50 percent from peak capacity. Enough.

If we were still living in an agrarian society, our lifestyles would presumably involve the equivalent of cross-training, but, of course, we would then not likely die of old age, rather of disease or accident. But living in a knowledge economy, we experience a sedentary lifestyle that correlates with increased education. Yes, there is a price you pay for everything.

WHAT TO DO? AND THE BENEFITS

If you drive to work or shopping and drive around looking for the parking space closest to where you need to go, may I suggest an attitude adjustment and just take the first space and walk from there? You may have heard that before. I know I shared that tip in 2004 and it seemed like a novel idea; now it is a common recommendation. But do you take it? The point is to look in the mirror and ask yourself if your normal daily routine involves at least thirty to sixty minutes of physical activity. If not, why not? Less is not healthy. Here's an instance where less is *not* more. Why are you living an unhealthy lifestyle?

Using our bodies will not stop the aging process, but it can slow it down... *beaucoup*. And we not only can add a proven year or more to our lives compared to those with a more sedentary lifestyle, but we can significantly increase the quality of our lives during our advancing years.

Physical activity can increase muscle mass and strength, increase metabolic rate, decrease bad cholesterol, decrease memory lapses, increase the quality of sleep, decrease blood pressure, decrease muscle stiffness, and increase mobility and balance. Need any more convincing?

When we think about using our bodies, we need to recognize:

- Strength
- Flexibility
- Aerobics
- Breathing

Your daily healthy lifestyle should involve body movements that will increase your strength, increase your heart rate, fill your lungs, stretch your muscles and connective tissues, and if not, you need to fill in the gaps. That means add an activity that addresses the weakness. Walking up three or four flights of stairs would seem to hit all bases. But there are times and situations when you indeed decide to "exercise."

Strength training is a likely candidate. The very good news is there are dramatically good results and benefits to muscle buildup, balance, posture, gait, and musculature via strength fitness throughout and especially late in life. So there may be some free weights in your future as well as the standard resistance training exercises. I have come to appreciate of late the supreme value of strengthening my core, and its value in maintaining balance, posture, breathing capacity, and avoiding back and other pains and increasing flexibility. So now I have tuned in to a regular series of Pilates movements in my weekly at-home, anti-aging or, rather, living-healthy-to-the-max campaign.

Generally, people do not injure themselves walking, taking

the stairs, or swimming. "Gym" exercises are something else. At some point you will need a trainer or physical therapist or to attend a class to help you select the right exercises that will address your particular body needs.

My husband has a short routine of morning exercises to stretch and strengthen muscles to address lower back issues. His exercises evolved a bit over a decade and recently a few preventive sessions with a physical therapist revealed that a couple of the exercises right out of classic exercise routines were exactly the wrong ones for him.

The Internet is incredible and can be a great resource that has made physicians and exercise therapists out of many. It is wonderful to be informed about causes, options, and treatments. It is also a dangerous thing, as we Internet-MDs are amateurs. Somewhere in solving our equations, we need the value of a trusted expert to work with, especially if we have any history of health issues or concerns.

THE MINIMALIST (IT USED TO BE ME)

Every Sunday morning when I walk through the Luxembourg Gardens near my home in Paris, I see a group of men and women, some quite elderly, doing Tai Chi. In the park, under the trees, this slow-motion choreographed movement is engaging and somewhat amusing to see. Is it exercise? Strength training? Balance fitness? Is it a leisure activity? Fun? For these people, no doubt all of the above. One hundred meters away, people are having their Sunday morning tennis matches. To me, both beat going to the gym. They are pleasurable lifestyle activities that are part of a healthy routine.

Walking is a part of being for most French women. We walk everywhere (at least those who are living *French Women Don't Get Fat* lives), and if we feel there is not enough of it, we create it. I see countless French women walking the stairs, not riding on escalators. I cannot say enough that walking is one of the best of exercises and movements, but too rarely do people in much of the world say, "I am going for a walk." Americans go hiking or work out on treadmills—again scheduling a workout rather than making it part of their routine movement. Really, all one needs to do is take a twenty-minute walk most days. Before breakfast is best, but anytime is good. Need a bit more of an unusual twist to motivate you? Try pole walking or aqua gym. They have caught the attention of the French. And then there is the universal approach: get a dog!

So let us be clear: walking at least twenty minutes a day is the very best nonexercise exercise you can do for your health and fitness. It is also the best weight-loss program. I do at least forty minutes of walking a day and some days, two hours. New York has subways, but on a nice day (and New York has comparatively good weather ten months a year), I plan to walk back the half hour or hour from wherever I am during the daytime. You can comfortably walk miles in that time. I have a friend who lives in Florida and meets her neighborhood girlfriends before work each weekday morning for their thirty-minute walk and talk. Excellent. Lots of benefits, and I am reminded of the old Mexican proverb: "Conversation is food for the soul." So walking and talking is soul food of more than one kind when we age with attitude.

I am simply amazed by people in apartment buildings who live on the second floor and take the elevator up and down. That is just about everyone in America. In my apartment building in Manhattan, it is not uncommon to see people, many in their twenties and thirties, take the elevator in their workout clothes to go to the gym in the building. I have yet to step into that gym . . . and I suspect they have yet to step into the perfectly clean, safe, and well-lit stairwell.

Again, a mirror question: Do you include this simplest and best of movements in your daily activities? One can start adding a walk to one's daily routine at any time. Certainly, in spring and fall in most places it is lovely to be outside, plus we absorb the light, which helps us mentally and physically. Again, a walking routine made up of a mix of warm-ups and stretching, cardiovascular effort (use a brisk pace for a while), muscle strengthening, and relaxation can do wonders.

I don't mean to suggest that everyone can fit all their exercise into routine activities; some must schedule a few or all times of exercise.

While working a normal business week, which for too many of us means long hours, the option to embrace physical activity can be a challenge. Personally, I added twenty minutes of yoga or a walk first thing in the morning before going to work each day (and more during the day on weekends). It became a religion.

Dr. Miracle (of *French Women Don't Get Fat*) gave me the best advice early on: whatever you do for twenty minutes or so, do it before breakfast. Except he never explained why, and young me never questioned him or thought about asking, "Why before breakfast?" My cousin, once a professional athlete, explained recently (he is in his fifties, fit as a fiddle, always in a good mood, and funny nonstop) that the method is ideal to shed a few pounds easily. (Yes, can I share a secret? I now strongly believe that twenty minutes or so of exercise or yoga before breakfast has allowed me to keep my weight steady throughout life.) He explained to me in simple terms that doing any sport before eating breakfast is a winner, as during the night, the body gets its energy from the reserve in fat and it continues when we get up as long as we have not eaten. Thereafter it takes energy from our recently ingested food. So try adding some movement before breakfast for a few months (don't forget a glass of water first, though), and watch your middle melt down.

If you can't get up early (or early enough) in the morning, though, don't give up. It still is better to do something in the evening or at lunchtime than to do nothing at all. But I didn't need to tell you that... or did I need to remind you?

BREATHING

The biggest discovery I have made as I have aged (here my self-conscious self wanted to write "matured," not "aged," but the mirror said "aged") is the power and importance of breathing. I am not being silly—of course we have to breathe to live. (We do it about 21,000 times a day as our body and cells require roughly 88 pounds of oxygen a day.) But breathing properly and incorporating breathing exercises and techniques into our day can be transformational. That is why I included it earlier on par with strength fitness, aerobic activity, and flexibility training.

Breathing can be all three and certainly is a branch of mental medicine. And as we age, the working of our diaphragm and expansion of the intake into our lungs adds oxygen that gives us more energy and endurance. It is an anti-aging attitude and movement that also makes us calmer, less affected by anxiety. Stress is not good for one's health, of course. Regular attention to our breathing literally improves our lives and health and our approach to aging. Why don't they teach that in schools?

In Provence, my husband and I came across a massage "therapist" from Cameroon who is a priestess of breathing. Her sessions are a bit like a séance with scented candles and a mantra-like slow chanting of "Respirez…respirez" (and sometimes "Abandonnez-vous" [Lose yourself]). It works…relaxes you in a hurry. (Breathe…pause…breathe.) "Respirez" has become something of an inside joke for us.

For years I was reminded that my breathing was shallow, and it was. I've worked to correct it—I am still working on it—and have made slow yet amazing improvements that have affected so many parts of my life.

I've witnessed poor breathing countless times in all sorts of locations and settings, watching people performing some kind of movement from aerobics to Tai Chi to dancing, but also watching people talk at meetings, make a presentation, or sing.

We think we know how to inhale and exhale and breathe through our nostrils, yet most of us don't do it well or even adequately. Watch an infant and you will see proper breathing, also called belly breathing, using the diaphragm (most of us breathe through our chests). Make it second nature and it will change your life. For one thing it will eliminate anxiety symptoms.

I learned about proper breathing and a host of breathing exercises through yoga. Yoga is not an invisible exercise; you have to carve out time for it. Yet apart from those who insist on squeezing as much as they can into the briefest of times... and breaking a sweat, it is a series of calming and relaxing stretches and postures.

Here is my yoga story: I had a class or two while a student in Paris. That's when the trend started. I didn't get it. So I forgot about it for almost two decades. Then in my late thirties and in New York, I suffered a backlash in a cab while on a job appointment, and for the following year the pain was constant (except for the hour at the chiropractor and the hour following), mostly brutal, and at times unbearable, until an Italian acquaintance who had lived here recommended her yoga teacher... two blocks from my office! Within two classes the pain was gone. Faith was the woman with the golden hands who did confess I may have to do some for the rest of my life. A new life, or my next life, as I felt so relieved, so happy, so overwhelmed that I could be myself again. I started practicing, first at her studio with thirty-minute private classes during my lunchtime, then in her small group evening class whenever I was in town. The more I learned, the more I loved it. After a few years, I started my own a.m. practice, and to this day can't live without it. It enriches my life physically, mentally, and professionally, and much, much more. When I skip it, I know my day won't be the same.

If you haven't yet tried yoga, it may be a good time to do so. It will add to your life in ways you can't imagine.

Some learn breathing techniques through playing a wind instrument and others through sports, including swimming. I am not much of an athlete, but I like swimming, even though I am not a strong swimmer. I paddle along. When I sync my breathing and movements and mind, I am shocked by how much my endurance improves. I just keep going lap after lap like I am walking. It's all in the breathing. So much is *all* about breathing. *Absolument.*

A nice thing about breathing exercises is that you can do them almost anywhere and anytime throughout the day. Here are four that I do regularly: The first is a simple and calming way to relearn breathing by focusing on your diaphragm. This one certainly builds up stomach/diaphragm muscles and has the bonus of flattening one's tummy and protecting one's back. Another especially builds aerobic capacity, and the last exercise calms one and reduces blood pressure. Amazing.

1. Diaphragm Practice

    You can do this standing, sitting on a chair, or lying down. Do it regularly for a few minutes and concentrate on nothing else. If thoughts come up, just recognize them, put them aside, and continue focusing on your breathing. I recognize that this and the other exercises are incredibly basic, but proven. Give it a try.

- Breathe into your diaphragm (feel your belly button go out then in with the tightening of your abdominal muscles).
- Think belly breathing like a baby and use the diaphragm, as noted earlier, because it's better than breathing through the chest. As you breathe in, place your hand on your belly and feel it expand with the intake of oxygen; as you breathe out, pull your belly button in toward your spine.
- Inhale through the nose and exhale through the mouth, taking more time to exhale than to inhale (you can slowly count to two for inhale and four for exhale).
- Progressively slow your breathing per minute (with deeper breaths counting to four for inhale and eight for exhale).

2. Body Release

This exercise helps dispel tension in the muscles and joints. Some yoga teachers always end with this session; others start and end with it. It's called "Savasana" and completely relaxes your body. Five to ten minutes is a good stretch. If you do it longer (especially at work!), watch, as you may get so relaxed you'll fall asleep (I plead guilty to that one). The idea is to stay awake, so focus.

When I am working hard or traveling and feel stressed, this simple routine gets me back to normal in little time.

Position your body correctly on the floor, lying preferably on a mat (I've done it at work on my office floor or when on the road on a hotel towel) on your back, which makes the spine relax. Before starting the breathing routine, check the following:

- Your head is straight, looking at the ceiling, and not tilted or rolling forward.
- Your neck is lengthened.
- Your shoulders are level/parallel and relaxing away from the neck.
- Your arms are resting slightly away from your body, with elbows slightly bent and palms up.
- Your hips are level/parallel.
- Your hips and knees are hip-width apart, parallel, with feet falling outward.
- Your pelvis is held in a way that maintains the normal concave curve of the lower back at the waist (until it becomes automatic, after the first time or two, this is the only part where you may need someone to tell you if you are positioned correctly—there should be a space between the floor and the curve of your back).

Now that you are comfortable on your back, close your eyes and mouth and start with a few breaths (remember to breathe with your diaphragm):

- Inhale slowly, pause one or two seconds, exhale slowly, and repeat for a few minutes until you feel relaxed.

3. Alternate Nostril Breathing

This is another classic exercise to improve breathing that you can do anywhere and anytime, even sitting at a desk or the kitchen table. I do it every morning and it brings great calm.

- To start, breathe through the left nostril. Close the right nostril with your thumb and inhale through the left nostril, counting to four. Exhale while counting to eight. Repeat six times. Do the same with the right nostril.
- When you are comfortable with the single-nostril breathing, you can do the alternate one. Try to do twelve rounds for best results.
- The next variation is to inhale through the left nostril while counting to four. Close nostrils and hold your breath, counting to sixteen. Exhale through the right nostril, counting to eight. Inhale through the right nostril, counting to four. Close both nostrils and hold your breath, counting to sixteen. Exhale through the left nostril, counting to eight. Do three repetitions and then do the reverse, starting with your right thumb on the right nostril.

4. Rapid Breathing

Known as "Kapalabhati," this basic rapid-breathing exercise is a powerful one, literally a cleanser. This one certainly builds stomach muscles, and, yes, breathing burns calories, but who's counting?

Find a comfortable sitting position. Make sure your spine is straight. To help you focus, put your hands in the yoga position: palms on your thighs and your index finger and thumb touching, and inwardly look at the so-called third eye between your eyebrows.

- With your mouth closed, eyes lowered or closed, do short, sharp exhales through the nose while squeezing/tightening the abdomen. Push, push, push air out your nostrils. Do not inhale; it will occur naturally.
- Start with twenty repetitions, then relax the abdomen, allowing the lungs to fill with air. You can build up to fifty or even one hundred repetitions.

There, don't you feel calm and relaxed?

7

WHY NOT REST AND RELAXATION . . . AND PLAY?

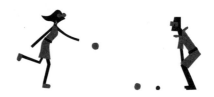

How many hours of sleep are you getting each night? Do you know if you are getting enough sleep? If so, how? What are the rituals you follow in preparing for sleep?

How about "beach" time (the mental and sometimes physical space where you spend time for yourself daily or periodically). The mind is its own place. Or *les vacances*? The French take their vacations very seriously. Do you? What's your idea of play? Okay, what's your other idea of play?

Sleep. Time for oneself. Vacation. Play. *C'est tout.*

The French, on average, sleep nine hours a day. That's considerably more than my fellow Americans, who seem to think it's a badge of honor to sleep five or six hours a night or even less. How many of you have heard, "I don't need much sleep"? Nonsense. Could there be a correlation between

French women's long life expectancies and their hours exercising their sleep muscles?

When in Paris, my American husband always notices the pitch-dark apartment buildings we pass while walking home late at night from a meal at a friend's house or the theater. It's barely 11 p.m., yet most of the lights are off. For one thing, the French don't watch much television (no staying up for late-night shows). They come home from work, prepare dinner, sit down to eat (that's entertainment!), and relax. Some may prolong the evening by reading or listening to music for half an hour, but by ten or eleven o'clock most of them are *au dodo*. No late-night e-mailing or typing away at the computer. How different that is from New York, the city that never sleeps! From our Manhattan windows, we see plenty of lights and people in buildings all around us until the wee hours. And the few times when we have to get up at the crack of dawn to catch an early flight, we are amazed to see those little lights on more than just here and there. Wow!

Of course I am not saying twenty-five-year-olds in Paris aren't out clubbing and dancing and drinking and making noise on the streets in popular neighborhoods on a Saturday night through midnight. Or that sixteen-year-olds stop texting at a prescribed hour...or that no one watches TV or everyone who does turns it off at 11 p.m. But compared with New York, Paris is on a different planet. In our Manhattan neighborhood, there are as many people on the street at 11 p.m. as there are at 11 a.m., probably more, seven days a week. There's no equivalent in France short of a train station.

Try these few tips so that you, too, can enjoy the benefits of a good night's sleep and you can do it naturally (the amount of over-the-counter sleep aids is increasing both in the United States and France...globalization is making us one size fits all!).

No matter your age bracket—forties, fifties, sixties, and up—the following will help you make a few changes; then you can tweak your personal challenge and improve your sleep and health (as the more one sleeps, the less one eats).

Move, move, move during the day! Studies have proven that exercise, in addition to burning calories, makes it easier to fall and stay asleep. No need to run a marathon or spend hours sweating; a twenty- to thirty-minute brisk walk or a yoga session will do the trick. (Just be careful not to do it too close to bedtime, which would have the opposite effect!)

Stay away from stimulants, such as caffeine, nicotine, and alcohol. All three substances make us jittery, interrupt our quality of sleep, and affect our ability to fall asleep. They can wake you up in the middle of the night even if you do nod off without difficulty. Many people who rely on caffeine to get them through the day are shocked to learn that it can have a stimulating effect for up to twelve hours after they've imbibed.

Try to go to bed and wake up at the same time every day. Our bodies crave balance, and if we train our bodies to fall asleep at a certain time and wake up at a certain time (even if we're still sleepy), they will eventually listen to our requests. No catching up on the weekend will change this.

However, after fifty, try to go to bed one hour earlier than usual twice a week and see how that translates to increased energy.

Reserve the bedroom for sleeping only. Okay, there's one other thing that is permitted—and it helps put you to sleep. But watching TV, balancing a checkbook, doing paperwork, eating, working on your laptop, or simply lounging in bed can cause problems when it's time to actually fall asleep.

Herbal teas work magic. Chamomile, anise, valerian, and fennel-blend teas are known to promote relaxation and help make sleep come easier. Most health food stores have their own specialty blends as well.

At my grandmother's farm, it was a half cup of fresh tepid milk and the house was in total silence for a good eight hours for all, age not a factor.

Turn off the lights earlier. Lights signal to our brains that it's daytime and can interfere with our bodies' ability to wind down for sleep.

Dimmers have a purpose besides saving electricity.

Turn off the computer and TV at least a half hour, but preferably an hour, before bedtime. Both tend to keep our minds active, the last thing we want before bedtime. Ever think the lights from computers can confuse our sleep patterns, suggesting day when it is night? It's true. I know turning the TV and the computer off is hard, but recognize that you need a little prep time for sleep. Now, foreplay is another thing.

If you can't sleep for a full half hour, get up and read a book (probably not of the action-adventure kind) or listen to soothing music for a little while. Staying in bed will only make you more restless.

Avoid having a very large meal before bedtime. Have your dinner at least two to three hours before you plan on going to sleep, and eat your protein for breakfast mostly, less for lunch, and even less for dinner. (I appreciate that the two-hour rule is hard when dining out with friends or family in a restaurant, but that's an exception, not the rule.) A light supper, starting with an evening soup (often done in French households), is conducive to a great night's sleep.

The saying "Qui dort dîne" (If you are hungry, go to sleep and it will replace a meal) works to a great extent: no need to go to bed starving, though trying to fall asleep and stay asleep when full or stuffed after that TV snack is definitely not ideal.

Create an environment that is conducive to sleep with a bedroom that's totally dark, well ventilated, and cool. If you don't have curtains that shade the light, try a sleeping mask. If you live on a busy street, try a fan, a "white noise" machine, or earplugs.

And remember: a bad night's rest/sleeping pattern means a short temper, a short attention span, more stress, and, for women especially, a greater risk of heart disease, not to mention skin that is not at its best. *Bonne nuit, mes amies!*

PLAGE DE TEMPS / BEACH TIME/ *LES VACANCES*

"Mon passe-temps favori, c'est laisser passer le temps, avoir du temps, prendre du temps, perdre mon temps, vivre à contretemps," said Françoise Sagan. (My favorite pastime is to let time go by, to have time, to take my time, to waste my time, to live out of time.)

As suggested at the beginning of this chapter, we need to maintain a mental and physical equilibrium to stay healthy. I am sure most of us realize that, but we sometimes lose focus on what's truly good for us. We need time for ourselves; we need playtime; we need vacation time; we need quiet time. Think of words such as *respite, refuel, restore, relax, recharge*, especially after fifty, when the immune system starts weakening.

Some people actually feel guilty when not working or when taking time for themselves. I'd say that calls for an attitude adjustment. The next time you meet someone, start with the question "What do you do for play?" You may be amazed at the look, silence, or admittance of their lack of playtime. Taking action to maintain mental and physical equilibrium qualifies as being productive.

That sort of productivity can take many shapes and forms. Playing golf, for example, takes a lot of time—so I am told—but obviously it has physical and mental benefits that keep people well into their seventies and eighties swinging away. It must be a nice feeling to smack a hard drive down the fairway that keeps people coming back for more.

Sometimes beach time is literally at the beach or at the

pool, and it is playtime. Swimming is an extremely popular physical activity in France. When I swim I certainly don't see it as exercise, but I know it's good for me.

Consider Michel Drucker, the French television host who has been around for so long some people joke that he comes with the purchase of a television set. Many French families watch his Sunday afternoon show, and today in his seventies he still looks and feels fifty. His magic pill: *natation* (swimming). We have an expression, "nager dans le bonheur" (literally to swim in happiness), for being overjoyed, and Monsieur Drucker certainly looks like he is having the time of his life. He became a passionate swimmer a bit over fifteen years ago and has convinced young and old in the entertainment field as well as among his fans to include swimming in their lives, and the number keeps growing. Doctors recommend swimming for the heart, the back, the morale, and the waistline. It is also good for worn-out joints, muscle tone, cardiac and respiratory functions, and flexibility. It also helps maintain high brain function.

For Drucker, it was stress and back pain that led him upon a friend's advice to start his two and a half hours of weekly practice. He was already an occasional walker and a passionate bike rider (still is) when in his beloved Provence (I have seen him around, and a serious biker he is, going up the steep winding roads in the Alpilles), but the swimming transformed him, not only curing his back after years of suffering but making him feel taller, as well as giving him a lean look and a young man's shoulders. He says that swimming saved his life, his abdominal muscles feel like concrete, and he leaves the pool filled with endorphins. How is that for a recipe for aging (or preparing for aging) with attitude?

PÉTANQUE

Tennis, like golf, is another recreational sport played long into life and popular in many of the world's developed and developing nations, including France in recent years; however, as a participatory sport, my French compatriots enjoy bicycling first and increasingly pétanque, a favorite of mine as it can be played with people of all abilities and, like golf, facilitates social communication. In France, a country of 65 million people, nearly 20 million play.

Pétanque until recently was played mostly in Provence and the South of France in general, as well as in Corsica and Spain (and, of course, in Italy, its close cousin is called boccie). Its popularity (and addiction) has spread in recent decades, and I had a hand in the 1990s in introducing pétanque tournaments around the United States to celebrate Bastille Day. Summer tourists from England and elsewhere have brought it back home, and it is common in such French outposts as Quebec, Vietnam, Cambodia, and Laos.

It is a team sport, with teams of two, three, or four persons taking turns against another in trying to place their metal balls closest to a small wooden ball called a *cochonnet*. There's plenty of skill levels and strategies, but pétanque can be enjoyed by children, novices, and modest (read dismal) athletes like me with joy equal to that of professionals. And it provides an occasion for a lot of beneficial socializing.

As a frequent visitor to and resident of Provence, I've seen it played by the old geezers in the villages since I was a child, including on Christmas Day! There are 570 clubs in Provence alone in the Ligue PACA de pétanque et jeu provençal, which has 50,000 members that cover six *départements*. I started playing it a bit as an adolescent and have not gotten bored by it yet, though I've never indulged daily like some of the men and women in my village. Lots of people play on weekends, including in the Luxembourg Gardens in Paris. It is also played in New York City, including in Washington Square Park, where I enjoy watching the regular teams play.

As I am writing this passage, it's August and a film called *Les Boulistes* (*boules* is a vernacular expression for pétanque) is being shot in my department (#13...named Bouches-du-Rhône) in the heart of Provence. The cast includes Gérard Depardieu. A series of sights in the area are being used as filming locations to show the diversity of Provençal locations and decor.

In my world of Provence, pétanque is often played late afternoon in the shade under the *platanes* or *mûriers sauvages* trees near the village center when the sun is no longer too, too hot (though often it is still sizzling). The game is an ideal predinner activity with the classic glass of pastis (with or without alcohol; count me without to see the ball and win the game). The game can be played on any relatively flat open space, though an official tournament court is called a *boulodrome* and is a rectangle at least 4 meters wide and 15 meters long. We had one built at our home. I love beating my husband, or if playing with him and a group, beating the other team(s). I get excited. And playing the game is free (unless you enter a tournament). By now, you've noticed that the French love what's *gratuit* (free) and what they can do at any time, anywhere (or almost), and without a special outfit. We are indeed born individualists.

We've had many games and teams over the years in our Provence home and enjoyed great laughter and happy times, but the most priceless one was last summer when we had an evening with about thirty guests from all over the world. It was my Japanese best friend Sachiko's first visit to Provence. She was curious to play but surely did not read the instruction sheet we had left in her room.

She arrived in a Hermès blouse and tight skirt with Loubou-tin shoes, and clearly did not have the slightest idea what this game was all about. But she certainly looked striking. You've got to admire and love that attitude. I'm not sure how she walked on the grass and pebbles before reaching the *boulodrome* when all the men and a few women were ready to start, and a few women were standing around watching, not yet sure whether to join in. But here came Sachiko, and as a good sport she offered to be on the first team. I would have liked to be in most players' heads to listen to what they were thinking. After watching for a few minutes, her turn came and she managed an uneventful toss and later others. But then at a decisive moment with the game on the line, her turn came up again. She positioned herself like a pro and with every pair of eyes looking at her, wow, she knocked all the guys' balls away and was the closest to the *cochonnet* and won the point. Now, if you don't know the game, this is a prize shot. With everybody overexcited and screaming, she quickly figured out that this was special. Yes, we laughed and celebrated, especially the women, with great French songs. It took Sachiko awhile to make sense of what she had accomplished and that her team had won as a result. It's one of the best aspects of pétanque: you may not play a lot or be great at it, but still every once in a while someone comes and shows you *zee* little miracle.

Pétanque won't burn the same calories as a jog or swim or bike ride or even a walk, but it is so much fun; as Baudelaire would have said, "L'art pour l'art," and here it was playing for playing, plus a great time to be together and enjoy conviviality. It takes one outdoors, is a hobby, provokes healthy laughter, and breeds pleasant social engagement and discourse, especially during those small intervals of picking up balls, waiting for someone to toss and start a new point. Also, some people behave strangely while playing. (I am notorious, especially when making a nice shot or winning a point or match, for becoming very silly and expressing my joy with strange sounds that can create a general giggly mood…Maybe I want to distract my opponents, says Edward—well, yes, it's part of the game, at least in my fashion.) Sociologists should study human nature on the court. Maybe they have.

Today more and more of the young generation is discovering and enjoying pétanque, and the *boule* industry has not lost any time in creating a modern version of the silver plain-looking ball and turning it into something trendy with vivid stripes of green or blue or any striking color. It is gaining much interest nowadays, with its popularity increasing at a rapid rate, and the pastime can be found in the most hidden corners of Alsace or Brittany.

No question, having active, social hobbies with their many benefits helps the "aging with attitude" process.

So golf, bridge (mental and social exercise), tennis, pétanque, or…What is your anti-aging diversion?

8

THE NONDIET ANTI-AGING NUTRITIONAL FORMULA

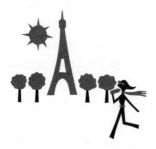

Think of a nice garden plant. What does it need most? Try water and sunlight. As women get older, they may think they need to take lots of vitamins and supplements to feel and look good. But before you worry about diet supplements, let's talk water and sunlight. As we get on in years, we need to pay special attention to both. Mirror, mirror, on the wall, am I getting outside and into the sun each day and not just getting sun through the light-altering glass of my office or living room window?

Want to live longer and healthier? Take a dose of sunlight each day, say, fifteen to thirty minutes. For one thing, sunlight signals skin cells to produce vitamin D, a vitamin or prohormone that many people lack as they age. Sad, as it is the least expensive medicine available to combat such concerns of old age as bone health and osteoporosis, as well as such dreads of any age as heart disease, depression, diabetes, and more.

Did you know that recent studies have shown that the aging of our eyes impacts our sleep and mental state of mind? Light—in this case the lack thereof—triggers melatonin, which has a lot of health benefits, including getting us calm and ready for sleep. Serotonin, a light-trigger hormone, gets us up in the morning with energy, alertness, and joie de vivre (I added the latter, as I doubt it has appeared in any scientific referred journal).

Rise and shine: studies have shown that bright light suppresses melatonin, so when our eyes age and absorb less light, blue wavelength in particular—oops—we lack the turn-on that gets us up and out of bed alert and in a good mood. One study showed that the stimulation we receive from light in our youth is down 50 percent by age forty-five and by seventy-five is only 17 percent. Wow. Turn on the lights. But lights don't compete with the sun, which is so much more powerful in boosting mood, helping us feel good, giving us energy, and triggering healthy reactions in our bodies after millennia of evolution and across the entire wave spectrum.

Could the French be living longer because they are still not a car culture like America and go out each morning into the daylight to buy their baguette? Well, many still do. Daylight is as important to sleep patterns and mood and physical health as water is to life. But who in this pressured life built on year-round indoor occupations recognizes that? The correlation between light deprivation and depression is well established. And who needs to feel down?

No question, as we age (or as we rise in the business world and work long hours), we often neglect a very basic need: to get out and into the sunlight. And as we get older, we tend to live more inside, where artificial "daylight" is a thousand or many thousands of times dimmer than the outdoors, and we put ourselves at risk for poor health and unhappiness. So, we need an attitude and discipline that says, "I am going out in the daylight daily." Tie that to a walk and a glass of water before and after your walk, and you have a remarkable formula for wellness that is often neglected.

Water is doubtless the least expensive anti-aging potion. And as we age, we can become seriously dehydrated if we do not "dose" ourselves with adequate and regular amounts of water. Water is one "medicine" where it is hard to take an overdose; it is possible, but nature has its own means of adjusting the balance.

The benefits of water are obvious. Our 100 trillion body cells (give or take a few) are—regardless of our size, shape, gender, or age—composed of mainly water. It is our number one essential element. Water passes essential nutrients throughout the body to all organs; it maintains body temperature; it removes the body's wastes and toxins; and it maintains the skin's moisture balance, keeping it elastic and soft (How's that for a low-cost, anti-aging beauty cream?).

For some reason, people have a tendency not to drink enough water when they age, and our thirst centers seem not to function as well as they did when we were young. But we also create artificial barriers, such as the worry that we will have to go to the bathroom a lot. Let us not be too vain or silly. Our bladders can adjust and be trained to handle the appropriate amount of water consumed in regular intervals. And an extra trip or two to the WC as we call it in France... *mon Dieu!* If you need an additional motivator, consider this: the brain has one of the body's highest concentrations of water, up to 85 percent. And if our brains become dehydrated (something we have all seen in the elderly), we become confused and disoriented.

But how much water is sufficient? What's the proper "dose"? The general rule of thumb is 8 glasses a day, or about 64 ounces (1.9 liters), which jibes with the Mayo Clinic and the Institute of Medicine's recommendations for women. As I wrote earlier, I make sure to have one glass of water *before* I go to bed and another glass first thing in the morning *before* I eat breakfast. I certainly drink some water in the late morning, late afternoon, and before dinner, partly not to fall into the trap of eating something or overeating because I think my body is saying it is hungry when it is really thirsty. But we aren't all the same size and don't have the same daily routines. I know what you are again thinking... trips to the WC, especially at night. Katie Couric asked me that on national TV when she was the host of the *Today Show*. As I told her, you would be surprised how much you can train your muscles and expand and accustom your bladder. It is just conditioning, then routine. Not a problem for most people. You get used to it.

Here are some caveats: bigger body, bigger dosage, but 80 percent of your daily water needs to come from pure water (with or preferably without bubbles). Coffee and alcohol not only don't count, but as diuretics, they call for increasing the dosage. So does exercise. If you exercise for a half hour and break a sweat, drink an additional eight-ounce glass afterward. Get an hour-long massage? Add another eight ounces. On a long airplane flight? Double up. In short, pay attention to your body's needs.

Another measure of the right dosage is one-half ounce a day for every pound of body weight (in metrics, the rule is kilos divided by thirty equals liters required). But again, ballpark, and use some common sense. If it is very hot and dry and you are perspiring, up the dosage. Ditto if you find you are getting muscle cramps.

Water is our daily and vital elimination agent, so if your urine is not very pale, that's a signal that you are not drinking enough water. Permit me to put in a plug here for the French weekend leek detox, which I described in *French Women Don't Get Fat* (and on p. 250) as a jump start to losing a few pounds and ridding oneself of those natural and artificial by-products of our twenty-first-century bodies. It is good for you. Eat the leeks for lunch and drink the soup. In that book, I talked about a twenty-four- to forty-eight-hour cleansing. In the "you can't get enough of a good thing" category, I read about a Hollywood-style two to three weeks of diet detox. It seems to me there's a nutritional balance disaster waiting to happen.

Water flushes one's daily excesses and wastes, which is essential to good health. So in a broad sense it removes toxins. Rule #1 again: drink your daily water. Periodically a forced detox using a diuretic, such as leek broth, is desirable for cleansing and rebalancing oneself. It is time-tested, and we surely have more artificial and other toxins to purge than ever before.

EXPANDING THE ANTI-AGING FORMULA:
THE PAINTER'S PALETTE

Okay, sun and water are two of the ingredients of the anti-diet, anti-aging formula. Add moderate but regular exercise (covered in a previous chapter), and now add proper nutrition and portion size to the formula. If you are forty-plus and are not following a good pattern... hello, time to change for your own sake!

Mirror, mirror, how many colors am I eating a day? Colors? Yes. If you are consistently eating monochromatic meals, especially in brown tones, you are probably depriving your body of essential nutrients. Thinking colors is an easy trick— at least for me—to ensure a balanced diet.

My personal rule is three colors on a plate and at least five colors a day. How's that for a formula?

Think fruits and vegetables, fish, meat, and poultry. Think carbohydrates, protein, and fat. Think water and wine and tea and coffee. Think chocolate. Think textures from soup, perhaps with *croûtons*, to ice cream, perhaps with nuts, to cereal to fish to red meat. Think variety and nonboring intake. Think a diet where nothing is restricted but everything is encouraged in moderation. At least three colors on a plate and five colors a day generally ensure a healthy variety of nutrients, fiber, and a ratio of carbohydrates, proteins, and fat.

In a world with too many people not eating enough fruits and vegetables, veggie and fruit smoothies are helping some people add (and drink) color—green, orange, red, for example—and balanced nutrients to a daily diet. Juicers and juice stores are a relatively recent growing phenomenon in America. Of course, eating the fruits and vegetables as fruits and vegetables is nature's best way of getting a quota or higher quota of vital nutrients.

Many government and health agencies publish recommended diet components, including variations of the "food pyramid." There are easily twenty-five versions of this from respected organizations, perhaps the two best known come from the World Health Organization (WHO) and the United States Department of Agriculture (USDA). No two are completely in sync, and all lag behind current diet and health research findings.

The USDA's food pyramid was introduced in 1992 but was significantly revised in 2005, and traded in for a plate in 2011, with fruits and vegetables taking up half the plate and grains and protein making up the other half, with vegetables and grains each dominating their respective halves.

Virtually all the food guidelines concentrate on these food groups: vegetables, fruits (including nuts), oils, dairy, and meat and beans.

But to give fish its due, we are better off thinking along the WHO's percentage lines of a balanced daily diet, consisting of 10 to 15 percent protein; 15 to 30 percent fat (most of the good kind); and 55 to 75 percent carbohydrates. For me, postmenopause, I think 30-20-50 (protein-fat-carbohydrates) is closer to the mark, but not over a meal or a day, but rather over a two-day period.

It is not so simple or easy to follow a nutritional formula or maintain balance; if it were, I would not need to write this sentence. People don't always understand the distinctions, and our bodies don't process some foods the same way, or in the same fashion at different times of day. Let's remember that age changes our nutritional needs, our digestive functions, and our metabolism, so ratios and formulas do not always fit precisely, and what works at one stage does not always work as well at the next. But it is important to respect basic guidelines and adjust from there. The French are not big into counting calories, but they do pay a lot of attention to nutrients and their quality and do derive more of their nutrients from fruits and vegetables than, for example, Americans. Me, too. And, of course, they eat their daily bread. At least in 2012, 85 percent did, and it was a prime source of their complex carbohydrates and fiber.

For me, this is clear: Eat with your head. Eat breakfast, three meals a day, or four smaller ones if you must, but the key is each should include carbs/proteins/fat...always. If you must snack, opt for a yogurt with a few slices of fruit, or a sliver of cheese with a whole wheat cracker. Past age forty-five, decrease meat intake, portions, and opt for quality over quantity. The junk food one eats when growing up does some heavy damage after thirty, so reserve chips and cupcakes and the like for indulgences. Ditto with wine: one glass a day gives you all the benefits. Understand portion size. Think of your fist as a portion, which is the common size and notion in France.

DELIVER US OUR DAILY BREAD OCCASIONALLY

It was a French man, a foodie philosopher in the nineteenth century named Brillat-Savarin, who first said, "We are what we eat." And it becomes truer and truer as we age.

Mirror, mirror, am I eating three meals a day? Am I skipping one meal and bingeing on another? Do I know what I am putting in my body? Am I snacking between meals? Am I eating when I am not hungry? Am I eating balanced, nutritious meals? Do I have "offenders" (foods that I OD on or that are not good for me)? Is what I eat adapted to my age and lifestyle?

As I grow older, I know that the more I learn, the more I know how much I don't know. I appreciate that it takes a lifetime for most of us to build our knowledge database and mental monitor when it comes to eating healthy and with pleasure. Ideally, it would be great to begin learning early with a great mother who knows about food, nutrition, cooking, and the effects of the bad food, including junk food, too much sugar and salt coming from processed food (and all that take-out food), as well as eating too much in restaurants. My Parisian friend Guillemette is trying to be such a mother to her young daughter, who does not eat processed food and started to learn to cook at age three. But not all of us are so lucky, so we must use our heads.

Restaurants, whether fast-food chains or fine restaurants, are border-zone dangerous. Chefs are not great masters at balance or nutrition and are notorious for extremes in salt and sugar, even when they use quality ingredients. It's the nature of the beast. You would think a preventive regimen would be mandatory in health and nutrition courses each term in cooking schools and medical schools! France is fast waking up to this.

I had to go back to childhood to remember why I am not a fan of snacks (besides the fact that when I eat three meals a day, I don't need one). Indeed, it was my mother who taught my brother and me, with subtleness, to avoid them. She'd say something like "You just had lunch," or "We are going to have dinner soon," or "Have a glass of water" and distract us from our nagging. It worked. While snacking was not really an option, the French sometimes take a small fourth meal called *goûter*, an occasional taste of something in the afternoon. We kids were granted this small bite after a long bike ride or some activity. Not a daily milk-and-cookies moment or a British afternoon tea, but an occasional nutritional pick-me-up, which I saw my parents partake of only on a holiday or weekend when we had visitors.

Breakfast should be the most important meal of the day at any age. Once people know why they need breakfast and the problems that can happen later when they compensate for not having it, change becomes easier. At home, Mom would prepare our simple breakfast way before we were up—going out to get fresh bread or baking on the weekend—and it was not a rush moment, though both she and my father had jobs. We would sit down to eat the typical French breakfast of those days, which may not have been the very best nutritionally, but surely had the inclusion of carbs/protein/fat: a slice of toast with a sliver of butter, a bit of jam, and coffee with milk. My parents had the same breakfast with an extra slice or two of bread. That was pretty much it during the week, but in those days, we kids had a midmorning glass of milk at school to sustain us till lunch, the main meal of the day.

My breakfast changed a lot when I started working in America. First, I needed the sustained energy, but also I discovered all sorts of good breakfast choices—including eggs—which we never had at the start of the day in France. Then I read and learned about all the options. At thirty I made some big changes in the way I ate, and again fine-tuned them at forty, fifty, and sixty.

For me, the daily bowl of cereal in my thirties gave place to a varied breakfast: basically yogurt for Monday, eggs for Tuesday, whole wheat toast and cheese with a half grapefruit for Wednesday, oatmeal for Thursday, and so on. Variety was key. Today, I have made more changes and savor my magical breakfast (yogurt with flaxseed oil, lemon juice, honey, and ground unsweetened whole wheat cereal with walnuts, as detailed in *The French Women Don't Get Fat Cookbook* and on p. 164) at least every other day, and certainly always if I have a meeting, lecture, yoga class, or anything besides my morning of writing, when I know that lunch will be at a regular time. As I have said, I always do twenty minutes of exercise or yoga before I eat breakfast. And I am still learning to eat slowly and breathe deeply—a constant challenge, as is simply and gently dealing with my limits and adapting to them.

Don't skip a meal, as you will risk lacking vitamins and minerals. If you really don't have the time to lunch or want to reduce your overall food intake, just have something with protein and a minimum of carbs and fat, such as a yogurt. Or what about a soup, generally a source of many good things including fiber? My aunt (Tante Berthe) used to say that warm soup feels like velvet in the stomach.

When dealing with holiday meals, beware the danger of confusing sensations of hunger with sensations of satiety. The risk is losing your inhibition and eating way more than normal, thus deregulating your system. Avoid the four-pound bonus at the year-end holiday. Indulge, but eat with your head and compensate over a few days. Again, put pleasure first; if something sounds or looks too good to resist, go ahead, take a deep breath, and forget guilt or anxiety, but be aware of your sensations of hunger/satiety. You don't have to overeat to enjoy. Sometimes just a few bites will satisfy your mental and physical hunger. Adding the pleasure factor and not denying yourself, but practicing moderation and balance, is a sure way to lose weight or at least to not gain any. For motivation, just imagine starting the new year at your normal weight or less. At moments of eating doubt, try to drink big glasses of sparkling water without too much salt in them (happily, big names such as San Pellegrino and Perrier have zero salt but some calcium)...and drink slowly.

FIVE POUNDS, FIVE POUNDS: THE BIG ALERT

When I was a high school exchange student outside Boston, I was introduced to the American Broadway musical. I particularly remember a satiric Elvis Presley–inspired show, *Bye*

Bye Birdie. There is one song, "What Did I Ever See in Him?" that begins with a doleful, slow recitation of the words *Eight Years...eight years.* I can still hear it playing in my head except it has been transformed to *Five pounds...five pounds.* It is a wake-up call. Menopause often is blamed for five or ten of those pounds.

Women generally gain about four to fifteen pounds (two to seven kilos) between the ages of forty and fifty-five. It doesn't happen overnight, of course, but gradually, though five pounds gained while on vacation or during the holidays and not lost can fast-track the gain. And it is easy to blame untamed menopausal emotions and missed sleep (from hot flashes) for eating chocolate or chips or afternoon snacking. It is well established that being overweight correlates to poor health and a shortened life. So, adapting the right food and lifestyle balance is an imperative to living healthier and longer.

Too many women don't realize the "five pounds alert." That's when it is essential to react and take the following action: for the next two to three weeks, decrease sugar and fat at the two main meals, have leaner meals than usual with veggies and two fruits a day, and try to do without wine during the week and just a glass during the weekend. It's a no-stress, minor-deprivation way to get back to normal. After five pounds and no action, you'll keep gaining, believe me; and it will become harder and take longer to rectify, so don't let that scale tip to the double-digit gain. As my Parisian friend Céline said to me, "After fifty, just looking in a pastry window could make you gain a pound or two!" I know exactly what she means, and I think it is true the world over.

For me this happened when visiting my family in eastern France back when I was a student or working in Paris. My mom would try to make all the dishes I liked during my stay (a survival kit of sorts!) and talk about those she did not make. Or later in life, after long travel periods with too much entertainment and hotel meals, I would also overindulge. When this kind of thing happens, I do my magical breakfast for five days that week, and for my lunch and dinner have fish or meat, two veggies, and a piece of fruit. No bread, wine, or sweets for much of the week is perfectly no stress, as I get my carbs from the honey at breakfast and the fruit at lunch and dinner. That's all. (Well, almost; for me, I have one or two squares of dark chocolate once or twice a week as a reward and to appease any thoughts of cravings. It is easy to stop at two, if you savor each fully.)

My other slim-down trick is to "eat like a baby." My favorite formula is to cook vegetables, like carrots: In a small saucepan, heat ½ teaspoon butter till it melts, then add 1 cup sliced carrots and cover with water. Cook till soft, then mash, add a few tablespoons of fresh orange juice, season to taste, and add 2 cups of water. Bring to a boil and add ¼ cup quinoa and half a teaspoon of a spice like curry powder or turmeric. Cook for 15 minutes, till the quinoa is soft. Sprinkle with your favorite herb (parsley for me). Veggies make food less calorie dense per serving, and this dish will fill you up. I find it the perfect lunch if I will be dining out that evening, or I like to have it for dinner when lunch is the main meal of the day. You can try it with squash, cauliflower, or any veggies you like. I like colors: red and green are tops. A teaspoon of crushed nuts can add texture and nutrients.

The main point is that you won't be hungry. Illusions work. Use and abuse them.

The other tricks are what we call *anti-gonflette* (anti-swelling), as many women get these pouches, unlike men's *brioches* (potbellies), but just as unattractive. *Gonflée* for a French woman is that unattractive state of getting fat unevenly in the waist area and a feeling of losing one's waist, thus abolishing belts, which is one of our favorite accessories, and having the whole belly area feel like being five months pregnant...or having a few Michelin tires between the breasts and the lower abdomen. Need I say more? Not seductive. In spite of all the excuses (like aging!), the fact is that weight gain is directly linked with what one eats, and overeating often comes from stress (which slows down transit). Stress provokes cortisol, the hormone that stimulates insulin, which in turn encourages stocking fats. In addition, when stressed, one eats faster, thus without sufficient chewing while consuming big mouthfuls, and at the same time swallowing air.

At fifty or sixty, there can be a lessening of stress for some at work (providing the economy cooperates), but there still are plenty of stressful situations that pile it on: the major stressors include the loss of a spouse, friend, or parent; an illness; or a big move to another house or state or country. Being stressed is not conducive to making changes, including what and how you eat. But instead of overeating as a reaction to stress, force yourself to turn to some other quick and diverting stress-busters. You know the usual suspects—perhaps pampering yourself with a good haircut or a massage, buying more shoes or clothes, taking in a movie with friends, or whatever gives you pleasure. But when it comes to eating, start making changes slowly and treat Monday as a page-turner, eating light (which does not mean eating "lite" food, which may have artificial and chemical ingredients, something I don't approve of) by skipping the bread and eating broiled fish with steamed veggies, while rewarding yourself with the fresh olive oil and lemon drizzled on them and lots of fresh herbs, which will easily compensate for other fatter ways of cooking. Enjoy a fruit by cutting it and eating it slowly. If this frustrates you, it's not a solution, but it's worth trying, as I feel it puts you in touch with what real food tastes like and helps you focus on the moment and relax. It's my take on a meditative meal. And you have heard this advice: get away from your desk or your computer when eating. The computer, fruits, and salads don't mix, a lesson many folks have not learned. Very un-French. I am also taken aback when I see people talking on the phone while eating a meal. Not much pleasure and satisfaction there.

What I am preaching is portion control of two kinds: one is what is on the plate; one is the portion (read size and shape) of your body. You have a reasonable amount of control over both. And controlling both adds good years to your life.

I am definitely against the fast fad diets that the French call *régime express*, as I see mostly negatives in them...except maybe the fast loss, but that does not stay long enough. It's proven that 80 to 85 percent of those who follow fad diets gain more back within five years. (That may seem like a long time, but it doesn't happen all in year four. Regained weight accumulates, and for many it is all back within twelve months.) Worse: their nutritional imbalance is scary and they hurt both the body and the morale. After fifty, it is imperative to go slowly to avoid muscular meltdown and bone demineralization. Crash and unbalanced diets can rob our bones and muscles of the very nutrients they need to keep our bodies sound. Use common sense. A main reason French (and some Italian) women don't get fat is that being gourmet and loving to cook are two great assets to losing weight or maintaining one's shape. It's not pure luck that French gastronomy is now part of the Patrimoine de l'humanité de l'Unesco.

Diets are addictive. Most women don't think about it or realize that the path of the first diet leads to more diets, and eventually you are addicted in the sense that you are always on a diet (how boring) or are seasonally on a plan to lose weight. Women acquire a voice that makes them feel guilty when eating, and so they take no pleasure from food when they eat. Like taking up tobacco, alcohol, or drugs, most women who start dieting never stop. Their lives are a series of unhappy episodes ranging from deprivation (while on the diet) to over-eating (when off and bingeing to compensate), which slowly but surely destroys precious metabolism. You should not feel guilty enjoying food, one of life's pleasures. The only nondiet diet is a lifestyle.

Diets are not limited to gimmicks like eating only grape-fruit, or eating only proteins or no carbs, or the thousand variations on the same theme that make the news on television shows and the media and lure a hoard of women into trying yet another way to lose weight fast no matter their age. Diets sometimes include all that powder stuff, the prepared meals, and/or products tied to the diet to make you spend more and feel like you are eating well. They often make you replace food with whatever product they offer that is enticing—some of it much worse than the most fattening of foods you would normally eat.

Today, even though you can have a doctor, author, or coach on the Internet help you lose those pounds, the myth and lies continue. You are simply following the same program as anybody on the fabricated diet, though it may be subtly packaged to make it sound like it is "individualized"; and your questions are answered for a fee by an office of so-called professionals, whom you have never met and who give you some basic answers you can probably find anywhere. That said, knowledge is powerful, and we can use a coach we know and trust or a partner to encourage, advise, accompany, and focus us along the way to eating well with pleasure.

The problem with the so-called popular diets is:

1. They don't work.
2. The weight is lost too fast (that's actually the hook to get you on it), as *fast* is the key word. Your body will never accept this and will get revenge and make you pay dearly for it, either by craving food and regaining lost weight quickly or by breaking your body down from the lack of essential nutrients so that you feel lousy.
3. You won't realize for a while the destruction diets wreak on your metabolism (make the analogy to a car, where instead of using oil you use water). Your sleep patterns can be affected, and your pulse and blood pressure can take a harmful turn as well. Lack of some

essential nutrients can impact the performance of a number of key organs.

4. And depending on the type and frequency of diets, you may get really sick and have all kinds of problems, even with your brain; as well as anemia, problems with your digestive organs, infections, fatigue, and even some cancers or other serious diseases that are more probable with a weak immune system.

5. Diets are addictive and make you lose basic food values, such as enjoying eating and sharing meals that contribute to a healthy body and mind.

6. Diets tend to be "one size fits all" (please don't believe those who say they are highly "individualized," as they are not), and that is probably the major mistake, as each of us is different genetically, physically, and psychologically, not to mention the other essential lifestyle issues from location to profession, eating habits, emotional state, temperament, and all that is included in the *bien dans sa peau* concept.

Women are especially the victims of diet trauma, as our culture calls for siren bodies... and many listen to the quickest tale and promise of the easiest path.

Clearly, many of us can eat whatever we want in our teens, twenties, and even thirties, if we are lucky. Then there comes the time when we need to face an aging metabolism that no longer responds to the toxins and excesses we are feeding it: our bodies start to cry for a break (read a recharged healthy lifestyle).

MEET MARIE-LAURE

My friend Marie-Laure was never typical of French women who don't get fat; she had been on one diet or another since her late twenties, when she got married and gained ten pounds in the first year. Over the years, and as her weight grew, she fluctuated with losing it all (for a few months), only to gain it back (for the greater part of the year). At fifty-four, she reached an all-time high (menopause and a couple of personal challenges did not help), with thirty-five pounds gained over less than three years (one would say sloughing toward obesity at the limit of overweight, in spite of her tall figure). She tried one more diet, this one by a famous French doctor who has been all the rage for a few years (the diet mainly appealing to French men who get fat), and in her case it turned out to be the final diet failure and signal that her body gave her before it was too late.

She ended up losing a bit more than thirty-five pounds, not only doing the prescribed diet but religiously buying all the products recommended. Yet within less than a year, all the weight was back and more. Out of desperation, she went to a *source thermale* or medical spa, and after her medical exam, the worried doctor asked her, "How much did you lose on this last program?" She replied, "Twenty-two hundred euros." The doctor couldn't help laughing, and to my friend's upset face he said, "Actually, we should cry."

The good news is that Marie-Laure's last big diet failure was a breakthrough milestone for her, and she changed her lifestyle to the commonsense one so many French women apply—in her case with the help of two stays at the spa and a truly individualized program overseen by a doctor and a nutritionist. She stopped "dieting" and embraced food in a new lifestyle approach. If you need help like Marie-Laure, and can afford it, do get it. It took her two years to get back to a normal weight, and she is still working on the maintenance. Now in her late fifties, she says she has never felt better, cooks at least five days a week, and has added pole walking and dance to her movement routine to great effect. Her appearance makes her "look" actually less than her real weight...she built up her muscles and is filled with energy and feels happy. To reconcile her feelings about food, she had to do quite a bit of writing down what she ate and her feelings about what she ate. She's never been so attractive and seductive and looking forward to happy times. So here is a trilogy: food/movement/know thyself. Again, these are important elements in my life and also in the lives of French women who don't get fat (and perhaps do not want or need facelifts).

Marie-Laure says she has one big regret: that she didn't change her approach to food sooner, at, say, age forty (a good age to start or restart), rather than keep trying quick-fix weight-loss diets for years. Prevention is always a good thing. We all know by now what we are going to face, more or less, at menopause, so I'd give a big *yes!* to sitting down in your forties and assessing your eating habits. Learning to cook, or growing your cooking skills and dealing with decreased portions are all natural and logical things to do before your body gives you the big signal as in a new and enlarged clothes size.

THE WALTZ THROUGH THE DECADES

One of women's biggest delusions seems to be that we can keep eating throughout our lives the way we did when we were young. The truth is a simple but nonnegotiable no, we can't. I know that I cannot eat or drink the way I could in my twenties and thirties, though sometimes my head forgets that.

For most of us, fifty is the age where we reassess how we live and eat, but it is even better to take measures to change our eating and exercise habits early on—small and intelligent ones that still allow for plenty of pleasures. We know and learn to juggle a few self-management issues.

Women in their forties should prepare themselves for menopause and the changes in metabolism the second half of their lives will bring.

Here's my wining-and-dining log: In my forties, I reduced meat consumption to no more than twice a week, and as a result increased my consumption of fish, which has become more widely available as fresh, nonfrozen. I appreciate that not everyone has easy access to fresh fish, but I always have had fish stores or fishmongers at hand in France and America, and I see them increasingly available wherever my travels take me. Oily fish such as herring, mackerel or sardines do not freeze well, and while fish such as salmon or haddock can be frozen, the quality deteriorates quickly. So if I can't eat fresh fish immediately, I buy it vacuum packed. And while I was always a big fruit and vegetable consumer, with the advent of more farmers' markets in America, I was able to increase my intake of locally grown seasonal fruits and vegetables.

I used to joke in my professional days working at Veuve Clicquot that it was a tough job, but someone had to drink all that champagne. In my forties, however, I could no longer tolerate champagne or other wines with both lunch and dinner, so I picked my battle: lunch was better, but more often than not my evening guests were more important, so I waited till dinner to drink, but carefully watched my intake, doing the old trick, which is to pretend to drink but merely sip… so when the restaurant staff comes around your glass is still too full for a refill. This is a good and easy technique, as your guests or hosts will most likely not notice. I have practiced the technique successfully hundreds of times. For some women in their forties, cutting out alcohol all together around menopause is in order and comes with no effort simply because drinking makes them feel ill.

By my fifties, I appreciated that I could no longer tolerate wine well at all, and gone were the days when I could share a bottle of wine with my husband or a friend over happy hour and dinner. *Reduce* became the key word. Three glasses on some days became two or one, and I had wine at only one meal (again, I entertained in restaurants for business reasons in those days, so was always obliged to have a glass of champagne. I cut back sharply at that time, and today don't have any wine obligations at all. On the contrary, wine is not a writer's friend). At home, my husband and I adopted the "half bottle with dinner" rule. We'd open a bottle, decant half of it into a half bottle, cork it, and set it aside for another night. Sharing a half bottle with our dinner seemed the right and healthy amount. And wine in moderation, as we have come to know, is healthy and anti-aging. But I practice consuming wine only when I am consuming food.

My food intake in my fifties remained balanced, though with my travel experiences and greater availability in markets, I added to the variety of what I ate. Embracing new foods and dishes is fun. However, the big change was in my attention to portion control. I had to watch my offenders: bread and dessert. There was a time when I could enjoy these in abundance . . . but not in my fifties. The food and wine challenge is at its hardest when we are out with friends, or at holidays, or when we are on vacation. At times, during vacation or prolonged visits from relatives or friends, I'd notice the differences and how mixing white and red wine, for example, was no longer a good option for me. On the rare occasion when a fancy meal meant that possible combination, I'd just pick one and felt much better. And for the first time in my life, I learned to split a dessert! One for two.

The sixties are more telling and less forgiving, I have found. We just don't need to eat the way our developed and commercial world seemingly wants us to, and we all know that most of us eat 10 to 30 percent more than what we need anyway. My portions are now smaller, and at restaurants I've learned to say "No dessert" without a pang of regret. Sometimes I order two appetizers rather than a large main course. I can live without drinking wine for a week or more with no problem, particularly if I am alone or with someone who does not drink either. Perhaps the most noticeable change since I "retired" from corporate life and responsibilities, and have much more control of my time and meals, is that I eat more vegetables than ever. I can live on steamed vegetables.

Last week, I had lunch in Paris with my friend Jeanine, age eighty. Single, a breast cancer survivor, she is, as always, slim and energetic, and something of a role model. She literally eats like a bird, that is, if birds liked soup. Every day she takes an hour-long walk (it helps to live in Paris). Whenever I see her, I feel like I am taking a refresher course on healthy habits for those of advanced years.

9

AN ANTI-AGING FOOD PRESCRIPTION

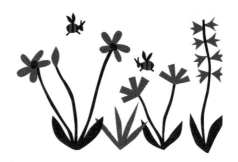

Consider that French, Spanish, and Italian women have some of the longest life expectancies in the world (eighty-four–plus). Also, consider that the average French, Italian, and Spanish woman does not like to break a sweat, though they keep active and walk a lot.

Science has proven that exercise and a good diet both add years to your life and make you feel and look much younger than you are. No news there. I could say, "The devil is in the details," though "God is in the details" fits as well. What constitutes meaningful, result-producing exercise? What is a good diet? There are lots of variations that qualify as good answers.

One good diet has moved beyond hype and is scientifically proven to be unquestionably healthy and not a fad. This diet is rich in omega-3 fatty oils from fish; rich in antioxidants, antihypertensives, and monounsaturated fats from olive oil; rich in antioxidants from fruit; and rich in fresh vegetables. It lives by the rule of a glass or two of wine a day. It doesn't involve calorie counting or banning chocolate, though fresh fruit is the preferred dessert. I am, of course, referring to the so-called Mediterranean diet.

Now think about the long life expectancy of those French, Italian, and Spanish women. The connection is not coincidental.

With some additions I have picked up around the globe, it is the diet that I for the most part follow. It is also the diet that the oldest recorded person ever to have lived followed, Jeanne Louise Calment, who spent her life in Arles, Provence, France, and died in 1997 at the age of 122 years.

But there are other places, cultures, and diets that have been scientifically linked to exceptionally healthy and long lives.

One such place is Okinawa, Japan, where life expectancy is very long indeed, evident from its large population of centenarians. Okinawa is a very socioeconomically modest island chain some four hundred miles south of the main islands of Japan. The culture is low stress, and the diet is distinctive. Besides eating a lot of leafy green/yellow vegetables, Okinawans eat surprisingly little fish and almost no eggs and dairy; sweet potatoes are their main starch, which have about half the calories of bread. Moreover, the Okinawans practice *Hara Hachi Bu*, the Confucian practice of eating only until 80 percent full. So they practice portion control. Net effect: Okinawans don't get fat and don't die young.

People have studied those Okinawans and compared them to their genetic Okinawan peers living abroad (and who practice the characteristically poor eating habits of the developed world). They have concluded that diet and culture—not genetics—are key to the centenarians' longevity. The traditional low-calorie diet of the Okinawans, however, has in the past few decades of globalization been evolving more toward the current higher-calorie practices of Japan and elsewhere.

Another documented long-living group, a group of Seventh-day Adventists living in Loma Linda, California, also demonstrate that healthy eating habits and lifestyle practiced for decades add years if not decades to one's lifetime. These vegetarians, who enjoy nuts, and an active and healthy lifestyle, live five to seven years longer than the rest of us generally good practitioners and are also healthier longer. They don't get fat either. Ikaria, a Greek island, and the Nuoro province of Sardinia are other enclaves of centenarians whose exceptional longevity is attributed to diet and lifestyle.

There are some obvious good guidelines for us as we age, as in eat more fruits and vegetables and don't pile on the calories, but there is other good news in the kitchen and on our plates.

IN THE KITCHEN AND ON OUR PLATES

So much has changed—and for the better—in the twenty-first-century approach to cooking. Today, we can eat well and better with many techniques and tips great chefs have developed, such as using less butter or sugar or even olive oil, and changing our cooking methods by replacing fats with stocks or juices. Or using less salt, especially on meat, by marinating it and tenderizing it. Or scoring meat to get rid of extra fat while cooking and using more herbs and spices for flavor compensation. Or perhaps using lemon juice in place of some of the olive oil or using grape-seed oil mixed with stock (whether veggie, fish, chicken, or beef stock, which all are easily available today and of good quality) in a salad dressing. And there's even a famous French chef who steams his veggies in a particular brand of sparkling water, which contains minerals that help melt the cellulose fibers in vegetables (thus assisting digestion while speeding the cooking time and keeping their color)!

For those who are still intimidated by cooking (again, a great activity and aid to knowing what you are putting in your body), one of my favorite chefs, Fred Anton of Le Pré Catalan in Paris, says, "Cooking is simple. It's either hot or cold, salted or not. There are criteria, techniques, but also creativity." *C'est tout.* I love experimenting. Another favorite chef, Yannick Alléno of Le Meurice in Paris, says when he cooks at home, he does not use machines except for his little robot (food processor), but does everything with his hands (nice stress-buster *et relaxant*) and uses only basic tools, like a whisk for beating his eggs. It's a great way to connect with food and to burn calories and tone a few muscles at the same time. No need for most fancy appliances. Use elbow grease to mix foods with a spoon, as French women who don't get fat have always done.

FOODS FOR FEELING BETTER

A few ingredients have been key in my life to provide me with stamina, well-being, and much more, at the least sharpening my taste buds, trying variations, and giving me lots of little pleasures. I also believe they have helped me age a tad better. My husband would replace "a tad" with "a lot," and I welcome that kind of compliment from him.

Those who know me and have tasted my simple dishes know that the ingredients I use most are lemon (and other citrus fruits, particularly grapefruit and orange juices, though I rarely consume these as pure juices alone to avoid the sugar rush and so as not to miss the benefits of the pulp or the slower release of nutrients when blended in a sauce or dish...plus, there are all those calories in a full glass); vinegar; yogurt and cheese in general (particularly fresh goat cheese, fresh ricotta, and, when in France, the magnificent, irreplaceable *faisselle*); eggs; grains (particularly quinoa, lentils, millet, and bulgur); mushrooms (any kind, and possibly with a glass of bubbly, the perfect accompaniment); fish (from oysters to mussels to salmon or any fish particularly prepared in the quick papillote style); potatoes (I am French, after all, and grew up eating a small portion daily—from boiled to mashed to roasted and, yes, French fries; but only on Sundays and no seconds, as plea bargaining did not work for children in our house); green veggies (particularly leeks, broccoli, zucchini, fennel, asparagus, kale, peas, cucumbers, and haricots verts (a variety of string bean); berries (particularly strawberries, raspberries, blueberries, cranberries, and including the almighty tomato); and, of course, nuts (particularly walnuts and almonds); herbs (parsley, basil, rosemary, thyme, and mint); spices (cinnamon, curry powder, turmeric, cumin); and the new fruits I discovered in my adult life, including avocado, kiwi, papaya, pomegranate, and mango when, alas, locally grown fruit is not an option, but I love to splurge on them and have incorporated them into my after-forty eating lifestyle. Of course, apples and pears have been my religion. *Et bien sûr, le chocolat, le bon pain et le vin. Cela va sans dire! Avec modération, s'il vous plaît.*

Most of the staples on that list stand out as super health foods. Here is *my* personal recommended and unranked top-ten list of superhealthy foods (it was hard to stop at ten):

- Oysters
- Blueberries
- Yogurt
- Lentils
- Spinach
- Quinoa
- Tomatoes
- Oatmeal
- Honey
- Apples

Perhaps the healthiest and greatest anti-aging food of all is honey. This has been so much a part of my daily life and nutrition since I was a baby I almost take it for granted, while it really needs trumpeting.

HONEY

Is honey a food or a medicine or a beauty product? All of the above, *bien sûr*. If you want to look younger and be healthier, definitely cut your sugar intake and look to honey. Sugar, which is hidden in most prepared foods, including restaurant dishes, and is the emollient of soft drinks, "refreshing drinks," and cocktails, not only adds to one's waistline, but it adds to one's wrinkles. High blood sugar levels cause glycation, which damages the collagen in our skin, *et voilà* wrinkles and the sagging effects of gravity from head to toe. And let us not consider artificial sweeteners, except to say, double your water intake to flush out those "toxins," *tout de suite*.

I rather like the notion of honey, as it is made from the nectar of flowers with the help of bees, so it is a somewhat "romantic" kind of food—sort of like eating flowers. My father kept beehives for some years, and the adventure and memory of "picking the honey" and eating the honeycomb add to the romance for me. Different flowers add different flavor overtones to the syrup, which is composed mainly of fructose and glucose (about 70 percent). My favorite is acacia, which is common in France, Italy, and China (and plentiful in Provence). Bergamot from Lorraine is a rare and special treat.

There are few empty calories in honey, unlike table sugar, or sucrose. You need a lot less honey (and thus less calories) than sucrose to sweeten your food and drinks. And if you are into sports drinks or pick-me-ups, consider that a spoon or two of honey in a glass of hot or cold water is perfection: the glucose provides an instant energy boost and the more slowly metabolized fructose a sustained follow-up.

Honey is just amazing: it is an antioxidant, antibacterial (it is an acid with a pH around 4, so it kills bacteria), antimicrobial, and has high osmolarity (which means it can draw water from things it is added to, which, as a medicine, kills by dehydration).

Its résumé as a medicine is long and distinguished. It is commonly known for helping with sore throats and coughs, asthma and hay fever, diarrhea and stomach ulcers; plus tooth and ear infections, pneumonia, cholera, scarlet fever... and on and on.

Its use in skin care and wound dressing is equally impressive. Records going back to 50 BC cite it as a topical treatment for sunburn and wounds. It has a remarkable property in that when applied to a wound, the honey surface attached to the wound turns to slow-released hydrogen peroxide, which is why it has been so successfully used for treating skin burns and diabetic foot ulcers. No stripping away bandages, just an easy dissolving of the honey.

And that is why it makes a great face mask. Just rub a teaspoon or two of honey on your face, leave for ten minutes, and wash it away. The honey cleanses, and its drying properties are an aid against oiliness, pimples, and even acne and some wounds. Yet it is moisturizing, soaking into your skin, nurturing aging skin. Wow. No wonder Cleopatra added milk and honey to her bath.

I had not realized until I wrote this chapter that I consume honey directly in some application at least five out of seven days a week, year after year, and have since childhood. Perhaps it is my anti-aging magic pill. (My mother used to say it would fill up my cheeks for old age.)

As I write this in my little Provence paradise, I am on a "red berries" cure (as in a sustained treatment of overdosing on one food for several days), including strawberries, raspberries, and cherries to beets to watermelon, and am eating them daily in different ways (I like Kerala pepper on them!). They are healthy, and a few days or even a week of indulging in them, especially when they are at their peak flavor, is not going to throw off your nutritional balance, but will enhance your pleasure. What I play with as time goes is a symphony of my favorite foods (well, perhaps a concerto), mostly from my childhood and late adulthood, and, *oui*, they turn out to be amazingly good for aging with style and attitude.

Our mothers and grandmothers may not have known much about nutrition, calories, or antioxidants, but they surely knew freshness, variety, balance, good taste, and pleasure. *Voilà. C'est tout.*

Here are some easy recipes with some of my favorite ingredients. They have been part of my nutritional plan since my fifties and some recipes since much earlier.

Magical Breakfast Redux

In Provence, when I have houseguests, I always include a big bowl of Magical Breakfast Redux on the counter buffet-style, and it keeps fine for twenty minutes. Because of its popularity, I alert my guests that a second bowl is waiting in the fridge, and more often than not, both bowls are empty when breakfast is over. Women, men, and kids all love the stuff.

SERVES 1

½ to ⅔ cup yogurt (or, if you are in France, *faisselle*)
1 teaspoon flaxseed oil (olive or other oil works, too)
Juice of 1 Meyer lemon
1 teaspoon honey
2 tablespoons raw old–fashioned oatmeal
2 teaspoons chopped walnuts

■   ■   ■   ᵒ■

1. Place the yogurt in a bowl and add oil. Mix well. Add lemon juice and mix well. Add honey and mix well. (It is important to add each ingredient one at a time and blend well to obtain a homogeneous mixture.)
2. Add the oatmeal and walnuts to the yogurt mixture and mix well. Serve at once.

I can't help pointing out how amazing this breakfast is because it is complete with balanced carbs, protein, and fats. The honey in it makes it "dessert," and we know that dessert at breakfast allows for maintaining lower levels of ghrelin (the hormone that stimulates appetite) and sustains higher levels of fullness. Plus, when you eat what you like, you decrease cravings. Lots of people think breakfast is important, but lots of people actually skip it. Surveys show that a good 22 percent of Americans skip breakfast, and among those who eat breakfast, at-home eaters are more likely to have a lower body mass. However, over 40 percent eat fruit and 30 percent eat cold cereal (Cheerios, anyone?) because it is fast. Not the best way to age well. After forty, a complete, what I refer to as "mature," breakfast is key: the Magical Breakfast Redux is one and is supereasy to make.

Beet Mille-Feuille (a Breadless Sandwich!) with Ricotta and Honey

SERVES 4

1 tablespoon honey

2 tablespoons sherry vinegar

3 tablespoons olive oil

1¼ cups (approximately 10 ounces) fresh, whole milk ricotta

4 medium red beets, roasted, peeled, and cut horizontally into ¼-inch slices

2 tablespoons minced fresh basil

Salt and freshly ground pepper

1. In a small bowl, whisk together the honey, sherry vinegar, and olive oil until smooth and season with salt and pepper. Place ricotta in another small bowl, season with salt and pepper, and whisk until light and smooth.

2. To assemble the mille-feuille, place 1 beet slice on a plate, cover with a neat layer of ricotta, and continue alternating layers (use 4 beet slices per serving). Place a dollop of ricotta on top of the mille-feuille, drizzle vinaigrette over and around, garnish with basil, and serve immediately.

Note: If golden beets are available, try using 2 red and 2 golden for a more colorful presentation.

Tartare of Cucumber and Tomatoes

SERVES 4

4 tablespoons fresh basil leaves

Juice of half a lemon

4 tablespoons sherry vinegar

3 tablespoons olive oil

2 cucumbers, washed, peeled, seeded, and cut into ¼-inch dice

2 large tomatoes, washed, seeded, and cut into ¼-inch dice

½ cup pine nuts, toasted

2 tablespoons golden raisins

Salt and freshly ground pepper

8 large lettuce leaves for serving, if using

. . . .

1. Stack basil leaves into a neat pile and roll them lengthwise tightly. Using a sharp knife, slice crosswise, creating thin "ribbons," and reserve.
2. In a medium bowl whisk together the basil, lemon juice, sherry vinegar, and olive oil. Season to taste and reserve.
3. Place the cucumber, tomatoes, pine nuts, and raisins in a bowl and stir to combine. Add the basil vinaigrette, reserving 2 tablespoons for serving, and mix well. Cover the bowl with plastic wrap and refrigerate for 1 hour before serving.
4. To serve, place 2 large lettuce leaves, if using, on each plate and spoon tartare on top. For a more sophisticated presentation, place a 3-inch ring mold in the center of each plate and spoon tartare into the mold, being careful to strain juices/

vinaigrette before placing in mold. Pat gently to compress and carefully remove ring mold. Garnish with additional basil ribbons, a sprinkle of salt, and a drizzle of remaining vinaigrette.

Lentils Three Ways: Soup, Side, & Salad

SERVES 4

1 teaspoon extra-virgin olive oil, plus additional for serving

2 garlic cloves, peeled and minced

1 shallot, peeled and minced

1 teaspoon fresh thyme (or rosemary)

10 ounces lentils (preferably the tiny green variety, Puy), washed and picked over

1 tablespoon curry powder

3¾ cups water

2 cups hot vegetable stock (if making as a soup)

Coarse salt and freshly ground pepper

Crème fraîche for garnishing soup (optional)

* * * *

1. Warm the olive oil in a heavy saucepan over medium heat. Add the garlic, shallot, and thyme, and sauté, stirring, until fragrant and softened, about 2 minutes.

2. Add the lentils, curry powder, and freshly ground pepper and cook, stirring, for 1 minute.

3. Add the water, increase heat to medium-high, and bring mixture to a boil. Lower heat, cover with lid, and simmer for 35 to 40 minutes.

4. To serve the lentils as a soup, add hot vegetable stock during the last 10 minutes of cooking. When lentils are tender, care-

fully transfer half of the mixture to a blender or food mill and puree until smooth and creamy. Return the pureed soup to the saucepan and stir to combine. This creates a creamy lentil soup with some texture. Season to taste and serve hot, garnished with a dollop of crème fraîche and a sprinkle of curry powder, if desired.

5. To serve the lentils as a side dish, drain any remaining water once the lentils are tender and place in a serving bowl. Season with coarse salt to taste and a drizzle of olive oil and serve immediately. You can add your favorite chopped fresh herbs as well.

Note: Any leftovers will make for a delicious salad over the next 2–3 days. Simply take the lentils out of the refrigerator 15 minutes before using and create a salad of your choice with some lettuce leaves, the lentils, and any other raw veggies you wish to add. If you would like to serve the salad as a main course or complete meal, 1 or 2 soft-boiled eggs are a lovely addition, as is a small can of tuna or sardines or some leftover cooked salmon.

Red Rice

Red rice from the Carmargue is available in specialty stores. I was introduced to it in the Carmargue, forty-five minutes from my home in Provence, as a superior alternative to regular white rice, and I find it crunchier and tastier.

SERVES 4

2 tablespoons olive oil
2 cups red rice

4 cloves garlic, peeled and crushed with the flat part of a
    wide knife
1 sprig fresh rosemary, leaves removed and finely chopped
6 cups water
Salt and freshly ground pepper

           ■   ■   ■   ■

1. Warm the olive oil in a large heavy saucepan over medium
   heat. Add the rice, garlic, and rosemary and cook, stirring
   until the grains are coated with oil and lightly toasted, about 2
   minutes.
2. Add water, increase heat to high, and bring to a boil. Reduce
   heat, cover, and simmer until al dente, stirring occasionally,
   about 35 minutes. Drain any excess water, remove crushed
   garlic cloves, and season generously with salt and freshly
   ground pepper. Serve immediately.

    This is delicious served with fish, chicken, or duck, or
made into a salad.

Skewers of Monkfish with
Avocado Coulis and Mango

SERVES 4

2 medium avocados
Juice of 2 lemons
½ to ¾ cup water
1 pound monkfish (swordfish works well, too)
1 large or 2 small ripe mangoes, peeled, pitted, and cut
    into ½-inch cubes

2 tablespoons olive oil
Salt and freshly ground pepper

* * * *

1. Cut each avocado in half and remove the pits. Spoon avocado pulp into a blender and add lemon juice and ½ cup water. Puree until smooth, adding a bit more water if necessary (up to ¾ cup water total). Season to taste and set aside.

2. Preheat a plancha (griddle) over medium heat or a gas grill to medium.

3. Rinse the fish, pat dry with a paper towel, and cut into 1-inch cubes. Thread 1 cube of fish on a skewer, followed by 1 cube of mango; repeat 2 more times on each skewer. Brush with olive oil and season to taste.

4. Place skewers on the plancha or grill and cook, turning them so that they cook evenly, until the fish is opaque and can be easily pierced by a knife, approximately 8–12 minutes. Serve immediately with the avocado coulis.

Zucchini and Yellow Squash Salad with Feta and Mint

SERVES 4

Juice of 1 lemon
3 tablespoons sherry vinegar
3 tablespoons olive oil
¾ cup crumbled feta cheese
½ cup fresh chopped mint leaves
2 zucchini

2 yellow squash
12 cherry tomatoes, halved
Salt and freshly ground pepper

■   ■   ■   ■

1. In a small bowl, whisk together the lemon juice, sherry vinegar, and olive oil. Season to taste and reserve. In another small bowl, combine the feta with one-third of the mint and reserve.
2. Wash the zucchini and yellow squash and trim ends. Cut one type crosswise into thin slices. Using a vegetable peeler, cut the other type into ribbons. Place both in a large bowl; add tomatoes, vinaigrette, and feta-mint mixture, and toss gently to combine. Season to taste and refrigerate, covered, for 1 hour.
3. To serve, toss salad and garnish with the remaining mint.

Poêlée of Mushrooms

Mushrooms from the "woods" (wild varieties) can be expensive, but are ever so tasty. You can, however, use the white variety and mix with a leftover boiled potato cut into small cubes or even a few pieces of bacon for added flavor.

SERVES 4

12 ounces assorted wild mushrooms (use a mixture of
    2 to 3 types, including shiitake, cremini, portobello,
    oyster, girolle)
2 garlic cloves, peeled
1 tablespoon olive oil
1 tablespoon dry vermouth (or white wine)

2 tablespoons chopped parsley
1 tablespoon chopped tarragon
2 tablespoons crème fraîche (or yogurt)
Salt and freshly ground pepper
4 slices day-old brioche or country bread

        ■   ■   ■   ■

1. Clean the mushrooms with a slightly damp paper towel, remove the ends, and slice. Mince 1 clove of garlic and set aside.
2. Heat the olive oil in a sauté pan over medium heat. Add the garlic and sauté until fragrant and softened, about 30 seconds. Add the mushrooms and cook until tender, stirring occasionally, about 10 minutes.
3. Add vermouth, 1 tablespoon of the parsley, and the tarragon and continue cooking, stirring, until most of the cooking liquid has evaporated, about 2 minutes. Add crème fraîche, stir to combine, and season to taste.
4. Meanwhile, toast the slices of bread. Slice the remaining garlic clove in half and rub the cut side over the toasted bread. Place 1 slice of bread on each plate and divide mushroom mixture evenly among the 4 slices. Garnish with the remaining chopped parsley and serve immediately.

Eggplant Caviar

SERVES 4

2 medium eggplants
6 garlic cloves, peeled and halved

¼ cup olive oil
1 teaspoon curry powder (cumin works well, too)
Pinch of paprika
Juice of half a lemon
Salt and freshly ground pepper

1. Preheat the oven to 350°F. Wash eggplants, slice lengthwise, and place on a baking sheet lined with aluminum foil (make sure the piece of foil is big enough to fold over the eggplant to create a "packet" for cooking).

2. Score the cut sides of eggplant with a knife and place garlic cloves in the incisions and drizzle with olive oil. Sprinkle with curry powder and paprika, season to taste, and cover with foil, sealing to create a packet.

3. Bake until the eggplant is tender, about 40 minutes. Carefully open foil and spoon the cooked flesh into a bowl and discard the skin. Add lemon juice, mash with a fork, and season to taste. Let cool and serve with toasted bread.

Sardines Sicilian-Style

I grew up eating sardine tartines—canned sardines nicely laid on small slices of bread. Maybe my mother knew something about antioxidants, as sardines are loaded with them, but it was not until early in my married life that I discovered fresh grilled sardines at a little restaurant on Sardinia's Costa Smeralda. It became our daily lunch, and since then I've made this simple dish often, especially as we can get plenty of fresh sardines in New York and Provence.

SERVES 4

1 tablespoon plus 1 teaspoon olive oil

4 fresh sardines (about 3–4 ounces each), cleaned, leaving heads and tails intact

1 garlic clove, peeled and finely chopped

1 shallot, peeled and finely chopped

1 tablespoon pine nuts, toasted

1 teaspoon sliced almonds

Juice of 1 lemon

4 tablespoons sherry vinegar

Salt and freshly ground pepper

1. Heat 1 tablespoon of the olive oil in a nonstick frying pan over medium heat and cook the sardines until golden, about 2–3 minutes per side. Remove from pan and place on a serving platter, lightly season with salt, and reserve.

2. Add the remaining 1 teaspoon olive oil to the same pan, then add the garlic and shallot and sauté over medium-low heat until fragrant, about 1 minute. Add the pine nuts, almonds, lemon juice, and sherry vinegar, and simmer, stirring, for about 1½ minutes. Season to taste.

3. Spoon vinegar mixture evenly over sardines and serve immediately.

To serve Sicilian-style, place sardines on top of vinegar mixture in pan and serve with slightly warm focaccia.

Provençal Goat Cheese and Grilled Vegetables Combo

SERVES 4

1 yellow pepper, cored and cut into 1-inch strips

1 red pepper, cored and cut into 1-inch strips

2 zucchini, cut in half crosswise, then cut lengthwise into ¼-inch slices

1 medium eggplant, cut crosswise into ¼-inch slices

4 tablespoons olive oil, plus additional for grill

1 garlic clove, peeled and finely chopped

Juice of half a lemon

4 ounces goat cheese, crumbled

1 tablespoon chopped fresh mint

Salt and freshly ground pepper

4 slices sourdough bread, toasted

■   ■   ■   ■

1. Preheat grill to medium-high heat. Place the peppers, zucchini, and eggplant in a large bowl and toss with 2 tablespoons of the olive oil and season to taste. Brush grill lightly with olive oil and grill vegetables, turning once, until just tender, about 10–12 minutes.

2. Meanwhile, whisk together the remaining 2 tablespoons olive oil, garlic, and lemon juice in a small bowl and season to taste.

3. Place grilled vegetables in a bowl, add olive oil–lemon juice mixture and goat cheese, and gently toss. Garnish with mint and serve warm or at room temperature with toasted bread.

Clams with Citrus Fruit and Arugula

SERVES 4

2 pink grapefruit
½ cup slivered almonds (or walnuts)
3 tablespoons plus 1 teaspoon olive oil
½ pound plus ½ cup arugula
24 littleneck clams, scrubbed
Juice of 1 lemon
Salt and freshly ground pepper

1. To prepare the grapefruit segments, cut slices off the top and bottom of the grapefruits and then slice away the peel and pith from the grapefruits, following the curve of the fruit. Working over a bowl and using a small sharp knife, cut between the membranes to release the segments and juice. Reserve 4 whole segments for garnish and chop the remaining. Add the almonds and 1 tablespoon of the olive oil to the chopped segments and season with pepper.

2. Heat 1 teaspoon of the olive oil in a nonstick pan over medium heat, add the ½ pound of arugula, and sauté just until it wilts, about 1 minute. Season with salt, remove from pan, finely chop, and divide among 4 shallow bowls.

3. Preheat grill to medium-high. Place the clams directly on the grill and grill without turning until they open, about 6–8 minutes.

4. Meanwhile, spoon grapefruit-almond mixture over arugula. In a small bowl, whisk together the remaining 2 tablespoons olive oil and lemon juice.

5. Carefully transfer the grilled clams to the bowls (discard any that did not open) and arrange on top of the arugula and grapefruit. Garnish each with the lemon juice–olive oil mixture, 1 whole grapefruit segment, and some of the remaining fresh arugula. Serve immediately.

Orecchiette with Green Beans, Potatoes, and Pesto

When my Piedmontese pal, who introduced me to this dish, is in Provence, she replaces the basil with fresh mint.

SERVES 4

1 tablespoon olive oil

6 ounces pesto

½ pound small, waxy potatoes, quartered

12 ounces orecchiette

6 ounces haricots verts

2 tablespoons chopped fresh basil

Salt and freshly ground pepper

1. In a small bowl, whisk together the olive oil and pesto and reserve.
2. Bring a large pot of salted water to a boil. Add the potatoes and orecchiette and cook for 8 minutes. Add the haricots verts to the pot, return to a boil, and continue cooking until the potatoes are tender and the orecchiette and haricots verts are al dente, about 3-4 additional minutes.

3. Reserve ½ cup of the cooking water, then drain the potatoes, orecchiette, and haricots verts and place in a large bowl. Add ¼ cup of the reserved cooking liquid to the pesto sauce, whisking, and then add the sauce to the potatoes, orecchiette, and haricots verts, tossing to combine. If the pasta seems a bit dry, add more of the cooking water. Season to taste, garnish with fresh basil, and serve immediately.

Duck with Caramelized Mango

SERVES 2

1 cup vegetable stock

1 whole star anise

2 tablespoons sugar

2 tablespoons water

2 tablespoons butter

1 ripe mango, peeled and cut into ¼-inch dice

1 cup celeriac, peeled and cut into ¼-inch sticks

2 6-ounce duck breasts

2 teaspoons five-spice powder

2 cups cleaned and sliced white mushrooms

1 tablespoon parsley, chopped

Salt and freshly ground pepper

1. Place the vegetable stock and star anise in a small saucepan and bring to a boil over medium-high heat. Simmer until thickened and reduced by half. Discard star anise and keep warm.

2. Combine the sugar and 2 tablespoons water in a small saucepan over medium-high heat, stirring until sugar dissolves.
   Bring to a boil and cook until the mixture starts to color.
   Gently swirl the pan to even out the color and prevent the
   sugar from burning. Continue to cook until mixture turns a
   light amber color. Be careful, because it will caramelize quite
   fast once it starts to color! Remove the saucepan from heat
   and carefully add the butter, swirling the pan to melt the butter. Add the mango and return to medium heat, stirring. The
   addition of the mango will cause the caramel to temporarily
   seize, but keep stirring until it melts and the mango starts
   to soften and release some juices, about 2 minutes. Remove
   from heat and keep warm.

3. Place the celeriac in a steamer insert set over simmering water
   and steam until al dente, about 10–15 minutes. Remove from
   heat, season to taste, and keep warm.

4. Score the skin of the duck breasts (so fat can render during
   cooking) diagonally at 1-inch intervals with a sharp knife to create a diamond pattern (be careful not to cut into the meat). Season with the five-spice powder, salt, and pepper, and set aside.

5. Heat a large sauté pan over medium heat and add the duck
   breasts, skin side down. Cook for 8 minutes, allowing the fat to
   render and the skin to become brown and crisp. Turn over and
   cook for an additional 3–4 minutes for medium-rare. Remove
   from the pan, cover, and let rest for 10 minutes.

6. Pour off all but 3 tablespoons of duck fat and add the mushrooms. Cook over medium heat, stirring, until golden, about 3
   minutes. Season to taste and reserve in a warm place.

7. To serve, divide mushrooms and celeriac between the 2 plates.
   Slice the duck breasts and fan out 1 on each plate. Spoon

mango over duck and then drizzle each with the reduced stock. Garnish with parsley and serve immediately.

Chocolate Soufflés with Piment d'Espelette

SERVES 4

1 tablespoon butter, softened
½ cup sugar, divided, plus 1 tablespoon for soufflé molds
6 ounces dark chocolate, chopped
¼ cup milk
2 tablespoons cocoa
2 teaspoons piment d'espelette (or paprika)
5 eggs, separated and at room temperature
Pinch of salt
Confectioners' sugar for garnish

■   ■   ■   ■

1. Lightly butter and sugar four 8-ounce soufflé molds and place in refrigerator until chilled. Preheat oven to 375°F.
2. Place chocolate and milk in a heatproof bowl set over gently simmering water and stir until smooth. Add ¼ cup of the sugar, the cocoa, piment d'espelette, and egg yolks, stirring until smooth. Remove from heat and set aside.
3. Beat the egg whites and a pinch of salt in a large bowl with an electric mixer at medium speed until frothy. Add the remaining ¼ cup sugar and beat on high until firm peaks form. Fold one-third of the egg whites into the chocolate mixture with a

spatula to lighten, and then gently fold in the remaining egg whites until blended. Place prepared molds on a baking sheet, and carefully spoon mixture into the molds so that each is about three-quarters full.

4. Place baking sheet in oven and bake until soufflés have risen and tops are just set, about 15 minutes. Remove from oven, dust with confectioners' sugar, and serve immediately.

10

LES SUPPLÉMENTS

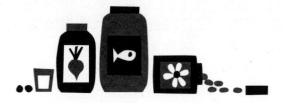

Pills. Pills of all kinds. We all want the magic, long-life, anti-aging pill. We are offered pills and more pills as supplements. There are vitamin-only shops that are panacea profferers right out of a Harry Potter book. There are big sections of over-the-counter supplements in pharmacies. There are big homeopathic treatment and supplement sections in health food stores (the one in my New York neighborhood has a separate adjacent pill store to accommodate them all). Magic diet and pill ads abound in magazines and online. I get confused. I get tempted. I know that many of these magic potions can do little good and many can do harm.

If you practice what I have been preaching, mostly all preventive medicine, and if you eat a balanced, healthy diet with good variety and colors, why would you need more of something that nature provides? With advancing years, you might, but of what?

The best thing to do about this in your fifties and beyond (if not sooner) is to get your physician to prescribe a blood test that measures a long list of vitamins and minerals. If you turn up with a deficiency, perhaps you first should tweak your eating habits a bit. A little low in magnesium? How about adding a banana (a magnesium magnet) twice a week before rushing to a heavy dose of multiple vitamins or a specialized magnesium concoction?

SUPPLEMENTS OF A VITAMIN AND
MINERAL KIND

Okay, a mild dose of a multivitamin probably will do you no harm and potentially a little good, especially if it is the new-generation variety designed for women only of a certain age. However, clinical study after clinical study has not produced evidence that taking multivitamins improves the health of an average person. They certainly do not cure any major diseases.

More alarming, however, is that study after study has shown that there are real risks from overdoses. All sorts of adverse effects may occur, and megadoses of, say, vitamins A, D, E, and K can interact negatively with some prescription drugs.

If you read the back of some vitamin, mineral, and supplement containers, you will often see the latest recommended daily amount from a government or research body. Then you see what percentage of that recommended amount is included in the pill or powder. And there are percentages like 250 percent, 500 percent, even 1,000 percent. Now who said ten times the recommended amount is ten times better for you . . . even twice as good? No one, not even the companies that produce them, and they don't because it isn't true, and there is paltry evidence to back up any claims that you will be healthier by taking them.

Also consider all the enriched milk, bread, pasta, and cereals we consume. They probably already bring us over the daily-recommended intake of various vitamins and minerals. Then add a megavitamin? You might set a day-in-day-out norm of 2,000 percent. And why must it be "mega" in our supersized world? You've heard that omega-3 oil is good for you and helps reduce the risk of heart attack, so you increase the amounts of oily fish you eat. Then you want to add fish-oil pills, which are yet to be proven they work? And perhaps throw in some herbs you've read about that come from a place and plant you've never heard of and a company you've never heard of, to pick up a little (is it cure or) protection you are thinking from something else?

Time for another reality check: it is safest to get your vitamins and minerals, your antioxidants and beyond, from fruits, vegetables, nuts and grains, dairy, fish, and meat.

But one of the fears of growing old is broken bones and osteoporosis, especially in women, so isn't a calcium supplement good medicine? At least that's what I ask myself when I should be asking a physician, especially the new class of physicians, gerontologists, who are most informed about the needs and latest practices associated with post-fifty patients. It is definitely important to get the right amount of daily calcium for our bones and more. From what I've read, calcium from food helps reduce heart attacks; supplements do not. However, it is equally important not to overdose on calcium. In fact, a recent study has found that women who consumed 1,400 milligrams or more of calcium a day had more than double the risk of death from heart disease, and if that is not enough, excessive calcium adds to the risk of kidney stones. Great. Have your bone density tested first, and ask your doctor. You may not need more calcium from supplements.

If exceptions prove the rule, let me return to vitamin D. I again confess, every few months it seems there's another study that comes out claiming that a certain food or vitamin is the key to our health, and I get confused. The media doesn't help, since every little study that proposes a "wonder" vitamin or nutrient or pill that promises better health gets its fifteen minutes of fame. But in the end, I come back to vitamin D, which just might be the supplement du jour to consider and reconsider.

This vitamin has gotten a lot of press claiming that many, many women are deficient in it. Now, again, for the average person, eating a correctly portioned diet that is richly diverse in whole foods (those are nutrient-rich, natural foods) will satisfy most of the body's nutrient needs. And if you go outdoors in the sunshine daily, you should get your boost of vitamin D. But perhaps only half as much as you think. Yes, ultraviolet sunrays on our skin cause a chemical reaction that tells our body to make vitamin D. But if you use sunscreen (and you should), or you live in a northern region where you don't see the sun every day, you're unfortunately blocking your body's ability to make the vitamin.

I stand by what I've always said and the French have always espoused: everything in moderation. But a little more vitamin D may well be an exception because more may simply be enough. And here's why. Although our bodies are usually quite efficient in extracting what we need from food, we do not adequately absorb enough calcium, the nutrient that is essential to grow and maintain bone and teeth health. That's where vitamin D comes in—it helps facilitate calcium absorption.

For years women have known that we face a much higher risk of osteoporosis and increased frailty as we age, especially when compared to men. To counterbalance this, many of us over the age of forty take between 500 and 600 milligrams of calcium twice a day for a total of 1,000 to 1,200 milligrams (our bodies cannot absorb the 1,200 milligrams all at once). (Again, more than this is overdosing, and it carries real dangers with it.) But this is what makes vitamin D so important: even if you are diligent in your calcium consumption, your body won't reap the benefits if you lack the tools to absorb the nutrients!

Why we might be deficient in vitamin D is interesting (and convincing); it is a vitamin not found in most foods. In many parts of the world we fortify our cereals, milk, and orange juice with it, but they do little in satisfying our recommended daily allowance (RDA). To give you perspective, most women need about 1,000 International Units (IU) of vitamin D per day just to meet their baseline recommendation. (I've seen very conflicting numbers on this, but 1,000 IU seems to be the median and 200 the minimum.) The amount in your cereal bowl? Only about 115 IU. Most fruits, vegetables, and meats contain modest amounts or none. Wild fish, like sockeye and Alaskan salmon, have about half a day's RDA, but let's face it, no one can eat salmon twice a day, every day. In addition to salmon, milk, OJ, and eggs are rich in vitamin D. It's not only food—or the lack thereof—that impedes our vitamin D intake, it is our twenty-first-century indoor lifestyle.

Today many calcium pills come with added D, too. So make sure to buy brands that contain at least 400 to 800 IU and specifically have vitamin D_3 (also known as cholecalciferol), the most potent vitamin D. Then you can get the rest from a balanced diet of good food and sunshine.

And while calcium absorption is essential to us women as we age, it's not the only reason to increase your D intake. Many medical studies have proffered that not getting enough vitamin D can raise your risk of breast, colon, and ovarian cancers. It's a major component of our immune systems— boosting respiratory health and reducing inflammation.

As we live longer (thanks to modern science), vitamin D is becoming increasingly important to the aging process. Deficiency in it can cause muscle weakness, aches, pains, and balance problems. In fact, people with low levels of vitamin D are three times more likely to have arthritis!

So, even if we have become accustomed to tuning out the latest health tip du jour, it seems that the vitamin D and calcium combo might be a notable exception worth paying attention to.

SUPPLEMENTS OF A HORMONE KIND

There is good news for us baby boomers. There is safety in numbers, and market and other conditions will generate more and more physicians devoted to helping us, and more and more companies researching and producing products that can help us. Some certainly do.

The most desired is a fountain-of-youth pill, but it is likely to be an injection or a cream. There are contenders already, but all come with significant dangers.

Estrogen, Progesterone, and Testosterone

As we know all too well, women's ovaries produce estrogen, progesterone, and testosterone (only about 10 percent of the amount in men), and the levels peak in our late teens, twenties, and thirties, then decline. Thus comes menopause in our forties or fifties, and along with it, besides the notorious hot flashes and sweats, comes a host of other changes. Loss of sex drive, vaginal dryness, and increased risk for stroke, heart disease, and bone injury.

For decades now, hormone replacement has been practiced to ease one through menopause and recapture a bit more of youth. Moderate estrogen treatments are often combined with the steroidal hormone progesterone, which helps to keep the uterus lubricated and stems atrophy. Together, the hormones boost energy, mood, sex drive, concentration, sleep, and even reduce the risk of some diseases such as heart disease and osteoporosis. However, attitudes toward this hormone therapy have changed in recent years, as some of the risks of long-term use—mildly increased chances for breast and uterine cancers, for example—outweigh the benefits for some. Hormone therapy is no longer recommended for disease prevention, including Alzheimer's, but short- or long-term use can still be a good choice as its benefits can be significant and a good risk-reward calculation for many.

That said, the jury for some is still out, especially on long-term usage. I am not a physician, and I don't want to make a recommendation or even comment now on all the issues, risks, and benefits. As a woman of my generation, I have had a good personal experience with this "supplement." However, I have also experienced changes in attitude, and when my gynecologist retired and I interviewed others, widely divergent attitudes had emerged among physicians who were not shy about giving their opinions. So study and learn, talk to a few physicians, and then make your own educated choice.

ESTROGEN AND *MOI*

Sometimes, you must decide what's best for you and go against the flow. As my mother would say, "Do go countercurrent... only dead fish follow the current," or, as I said in my business book, "Don't be afraid to take calculated risks."

Sometimes risk-taking involves a lot of weighing the pros and cons and then making the decision, aware of the potential risks and being ready to swallow the consequences. At age fifty, that infamous magic number that says "menopause phase," I was being asked (at least as a French woman thinking, *Life starts at fifty*) to take risks with my health, a first and quite different thing from taking business risks!

At the time, I was CEO of Clicquot Inc., which meant long days, six days a week, lots of travel, jet lag, stress from all the joys and pains of growing the company, and more. No need to tell you that my first sweaty night was ill received, to say the least. I had heard countless stories of the suffering of women colleagues, and I was not ready to live with the physical impediments of menopause, night or day. For the time it was night only. Unpleasant, to put it mildly. *Insupportable* (unbearable) for no-nonsense *moi*.

I visited my gynecologist, a New York pro who was born and educated in Greece. At our first meetings he intimidated me by always starting the visit with a "So, how is your sex life?" No question he was a fully assimilated American. That would never happen in France. But he had seen and heard it all, and seeing my *It's none of your business* look, he'd say, "You look like a woman *bien dans sa peau* . . . just checking" (he spoke French), and from then on we became pals and could joke easily about life, women, and, *oui*, sex.

At my first menopause visit, he recommended, rightly so it seems to me, a combo of estrogen and progesterone . . . with the pluses and minuses of taking the supplements all well described. And so I went for it, but quickly didn't feel right, though the hot flashes vanished almost instantly. He felt it was the progesterone my body didn't like (made sense to me), and although it's usually not recommended to go estrogen solo, that's what I picked, and his answer was "As long as we do a regular check with a sonogram, it's okay." (He was also an obstetrician and could take the sonogram in his office as part of the visit.) And from that day on, I once again felt terrific, physically, emotionally, and sexually.

But then, as happens regularly these days and confuses so many women, some risks were revealed through yet another study. And risks associated with the dangers of hormone therapy got doctors in the United States scared of being sued or of being accused of practicing "bad" medicine. So my doctor announced my estrogen plan would have to be nixed. "Impossible," I said, as a stubborn French woman. Not for me. I told him I would bear the responsibilities and would sign anything to cover him, and so he agreed to let me continue the small dose of estrogen. In my pseudo-medical mind, I still don't understand why we don't all take a tiny bit of estrogen after fifty since we need it and don't produce it anymore, but hey, what do I know? The fact was and is that I've never felt better.

An amusing development was that by the following year, he mentioned that I must be doing something right, as my bill of health was great and many of his patients felt lousy and were ready to go back to whatever therapy they had been on before the put-on-the-brakes study. Like me, they were ready to assume the risks. And in all my years with him and estrogen, only once did the sonogram turn up something (which, after a month off estrogen, disappeared). Many of his patients and I decided to pick what allowed us to live a normal life because all the side effects of menopause just did not make for a "quality of life" we were willing to bear (or inflict upon others). For me it was well worth the price of admission.

But my drama was not over. My gynecologist, getting on in years, retired and pointed out it would be hard to find another gynecologist who would agree to keep me on estrogen (though the dose had been reduced and reduced and was now close to the absolute minimum), and eventually (like soon!) I should get off. That's when I told him the story of my aunt Mireille, who lives in the Ardèche in France and at eighty-five is still taking some estrogen . . . and looks and feels like a woman of fifty or sixty (her daughter confirms it). He was not surprised and just looked at me and said, "Ah, the Mireilles of the world, a heck of a womankind," whatever that meant. It was the last time I saw him. And I should point out I am not being reckless.

The new gynecologist I now see is definitely not a Dr. Miracle type. After a lot of "discussions," she lets me use estrogen, though she has been tweaking with the tiny yearly reduction of the dose in order to eventually get me off it, as she claims it's mostly for osteoporosis and at this point in my life has no effect. I don't believe her, and as of this writing we are at a point where I am unwilling to give up the speck of a dose completely. Why? you may ask. Because I just feel terrific and attribute it rightly or wrongly to the tiny dose of estrogen. Who knows how long she'll let me stay on it or if I'll be willing to change doctors once more to find one who is willing to let me continue on it. Plus, I recently consulted a gynecological oncologist who assured me a trace of estrogen is common and safe, and he has seen a ninety-five-year-old taking it. So, for now all is well with me . . . going against the current.

Testosterone

With a much shorter history and database of users, the addition of testosterone to the anti-aging arsenal is a bit risky and controversial. Another hormonal steroid, it generally produces an improved sense of well-being and a significantly improved sex drive. It augments the benefits of estrogen and progesterone when needed and may reduce the risk of certain diseases, but it has some undesirable side effects. And while it may be invaluable for many patients, it is a prescription drug that requires close monitoring by physicians and regular blood testing.

Also of note is that while testosterone may be part of a "Hollywood-style cure" for aging, beware from whom you seek advice and receive information (i.e., celebrities). But mostly understand that there is an emerging class of anti-aging physicians who are a subset of gerontologists, who have drunk the Kool-Aid, are true believers, and are aggressive in their recommendations (which, of course, are coincidentally in their own best financial interests). If you go to a house painter, you will get your house painted. If you go to an anti-aging physician, you will likely get hormone-replacement recommendations. I am no physician and think it may be best to wait and see more of the results of studies on this supplement.

Human Growth Hormone

Now we are really into the latest magic needle of aging celebrities…and a dream of eternal youth. Human growth hormone (HGH), designed as a treatment for stunted childhood growth and hormonal deficiency, is, of course, a powerful steroid, banned among athletes in most sports. It is not certified, nor has it been studied much as an anti-aging treatment for mature adults.

HGH is controversial. The claims are that it reduces body fat and enhances muscle tone and bulk, boosts sexual performance, firms one's skin, and heightens one's mood. The evidence among athletes and black market sales bear some witness to this.

However, the long-term effects are severely suspect and include heart disease and diabetes, and the medical community is clear that short-term risks of carpal tunnel syndrome, joint and muscle pain, and swelling of the arms and legs are real and significant.

What is also clear is that the list of what I might call rejuvenation medicines will grow longer, clearer, and better defined and detailed in the next few decades. But what I have learned over the last few decades is that there is a price to be paid for everything.

Aging is a natural process, and it is delusional to think that simply bringing hormone levels back to what they were at age twenty will turn the full body's look and health back to one's physical prime. Or not have consequences. I am not being delusional about taking a speck of estrogen or a periodic dose of vitamin D. Stay tuned: the risk-rewards game will only become clearer and more dramatic with the advances and challenges science will bring. But for now, each winter for six weeks I will continue to take what has worked for years at my hairstylist's recommendation: a Nutricap supplement (from the US company of that name with a big global presence, notably in England and France), which is a pill, containing gelatin, walnut oil, carob, and lecithin, that is good for my hair and nails...until, of course, a definitive study of any sad consequences in mice appears.

11

LIFE EXPECTANCY—LIVING TO ONE HUNDRED?!

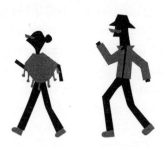

Do you want to live to be one hundred? Really? Most people surveyed today think eighty or thereabouts would be good, but increasing numbers are thinking a healthy one hundred would be nice. And you? It might be time to recalculate your age and to think about what medical science can fix. In America, more and more people are buying longevity insurance, annuities that start paying out monthly at age eighty-five!

If you have ever been to a school reunion after many years or some organized gathering of longtime friends or relatives, like I have, you will no doubt have said to yourself, *So-and-so looks really good*, and *So-and-so looks . . . well . . .* People the same age often do not appear to be the same age, and it is always flattering when people think we are younger than we are. There comes a time in life when genetics and environment take their toll; some people age well and slowly, some not so well.

There is mental age, which is an attitude, and it is something we can work on improving effectively. Then there is physical appearance, which we have a reasonable amount of control over in looking our age or a bit less, from choosing our clothes to how our hair looks to controlling our weight, to using cosmetics and perhaps cosmetic surgery. Disposable income helps here.

But then there is the state of our insides, our true physical age. Some of our parts simply wear out and show their age. Up till now in this book, I have focused mostly on preventive measures and anti-aging practices that will help to keep our machines working well, our appearances looking good, and our souls feeling well for as long as practical. We have now entered the post-genome period, and over the next half century there will be a "restorative" focus on what science and technology can do to help us live well longer. Bring on the regenerative organs and replacement parts.

LIFE EXPECTANCY AND *LIFE* EXPECTANCY

How do you measure up at your class reunions? How do you measure up physically? How long will you live?

Would you like to know today the age at which you will pass on? If you did, what would you do differently, or perhaps what would you have liked to have done differently?

We know more today about life expectancy than we have

ever known. What about yours? At some point in life, when we begin to seriously contemplate retirement, we unofficially shift our focus from our chronological age in years to a life expectancy, the number of years till we die. It is a sobering moment.

Two of the most common worries people growing old today have is *Who will take care of me?*, and *Will I have enough money to support myself till I die?* In the developed world and in the new era of globalization where children often live and work far from their parents, the old practice of children becoming their parents' parents is diminishing and is often simply not possible. This is true in the United States, in France, in China…in most places. It is a worry for many. Plus, for parents who have been their parents' parents at some point, they don't want to burden their own children, and they want to enjoy the lifestyle they prefer for their final years. I have heard people say, "I want to die of a heart attack at age ninety in the beauty parlor." Or "I want to die on the day that I have spent my last penny."

Nowadays, with people's increasing longevity, many nations have set up social security networks for health and retirement, but their cost and sufficiency are a daily worry of individuals and nations.

In the United States, the safety-net government-provided retirement system, Social Security, was established in 1935, and the first monthly payments began in 1940. It provided that at age sixty-five, when you retired from work, you would receive (including a spouse) a reasonable monthly sum to live modestly for the rest of your years. At that time, though, the average life expectancy for Americans at birth was less than sixty-five. Today it is about age seventy-nine overall and eighty-two for women in America...and the system is slowly going broke. Life expectancy in France is 81.5 years for men and women, but for women only today at birth it is 85.3 years. However, there is more to life expectancy (which I will get to in a moment), and for those who reached retirement age in America in 1940, they enjoyed the benefit for thirteen years or so.

I have a friend, Pamela, age sixty, who told me last week that she had always expected to retire at age sixty-five, which was and is a standard, unquestioned number and target in America, implanted at birth it seems. But she read a mention in a publication about the probability of her living to ninety, and she realized, "I don't want to be retired that long, and I cannot afford to be retired that long." She reset her retirement clock to seventy.

Average life expectancy is a frequently used but also misleading and surprisingly misunderstood number. Not only is it a composite number averaging a lot of people from different backgrounds and conditions, it averages men and women (and women live longer), and, most significantly, it is a count from birth. Once one survives infant mortality factors, the average age expectancy goes up. In effect, for each year you are alive, the average life expectancy in your country or group goes up, with you included.

Also, note the word *average*. Today, as mentioned above, if a girl is born in France, she is, on average, expected to live to the age of eighty-five. But that means that she has a *50 percent chance of living beyond eighty-five*. If you reach sixty-five, the percentage chance for your living beyond eighty-five is much, much higher than at birth or at age twenty-one. Throw in some individualized factors such as health, education, genetics, and race (whites have the highest life expectancy), and you can anticipate an even longer life expectancy.

Based on some reliable data, and assumptions and interpolations I've made, I believe it is safe to say that *if you are reading this book, you have a 1 in 10 chance of living to ninety-five years of age or beyond!*

Who wants to live till ninety-five if the last five years are spent in pain not pleasure, or, as we fear today, if we won't even remember who we are for the last five years?

Insurance companies, annuity and pension funds, and government social security plans all play the game of averages, including regarding our health needs. The half who don't make it to the average age help pay for the half who do.

If you want to age with attitude, many averages, especially the average life expectancy at birth, are not sufficiently helpful. The two expectancies you should be interested in are (1) your own current life expectancy, sometimes restated as your "remaining life expectancy," and (2) your remaining years of healthful life expectancy.

The European Commission has become interested in healthy life years (HLY), which is a complementary form of life expectancy related to quality of life and years without chronic diseases. For all of us now, I believe the most helpful published statistics are the estimates of average life expectancy at age sixty-five (or, if available, at your current age) versus the broader life expectancy at birth.

So, for example, in the United States the average life expectancy at birth for women is 81.1 years, but if you are now sixty-five, it is 85.4 for you. That means half of those age sixty-five will reach eighty-five, and half will live *longer* than that.

WHAT ABOUT ME?

Average statistics are useful for benchmarking and planning, especially when dealing with populations of significant size. But most are interested in a population of one: Myself. *Moi.*

One sort of rule-of-thumb life-expectancy calculator is the speed and agility of your walking at age seventy-five. If you walk like someone half your age or thereabout...add ten years. You can expect to live to at least eighty-five.

There are increasing numbers of personalized life-expectancy calculators available on the Web at no or modest cost. Just go to a search engine and find a few, and you are in for an interesting exercise. Take ten minutes of answering simple questions about yourself—your sex, age, height, and weight; your marital status and your network of friends; your lifestyle as it relates to stress and to healthy habits, or rather unhealthy habits, such as smoking and eating poorly, or healthy and frequent mental and physical activity and exercise; your medical condition, from blood pressure and cholesterol level to history of disease and chronic conditions to your family's medical history—then press return *et voilà*: your estimated life expectancy appears.

I tried it. I think I must have lied about all the chocolate I eat...underestimating *un petit peu*. The number that came up was 104 years. Yikes!

I don't believe it, but I am normal weight, I eat exceptionally healthy, my blood pressure and cholesterol are more than good, I walk and do yoga every day, my family has no history of heart attacks or cancer, and my mother lived to age ninety-six. As I said, yikes. Even if I shave ten years off the estimate for "cheating by giving upbeat answers on the test," or for being on the low side of average, or for the test not being all that it should be, and perhaps having a wide margin of error...still, still...living healthy for a long time is certainly the goal and guides the decisions I make now.

Thankfully, science and technology are already helping a lot. We should be able to live healthier and function better and happier longer than those who have come before us.

BIONICALLY YOURS

Do you not know someone who has had his or her knee or knees replaced? Replacement parts are in, and essentially only a generation old and improving daily. Jane Fonda, the famed, attractive actress and best-selling health-and-exercise-book pundit born in 1937, has an artificial knee, hip, and some vertebrae.

I haven't had to replace many parts yet—just a couple of tooth implants that work well, thank you very much—but if transplants and implants improve one's quality of life and let the inner self shine through, so much the better for living today. Maybe eighty-five or ninety can be met head-on and be the new seventy-five? (Hey, a positive mind-set alone is supposedly good for adding ten years.)

The French have very good doctors and advanced medicine (as well as the health-care costs and cuts many nations face today), and while not so inclined as Americans to invasive actions, certainly the French are aware of options, and in our anti-aging plans to live longer and healthy, we need to recognize their place. So, while I am no physician, let me do a quick run-through of what we have to consider in our aging-with-attitude approach to life. Here is how science and technology provide prescriptive, not preventive medicine; let us count some of the ways... but only the ways that approximate normal function and support healthy life years (not science fiction).

Eyes: The eyes are the first to go, right? Yes, at around forty, many people's arms suddenly seem too short or letters too small. Glasses have been around for centuries, but none so effective as today's computer-generated laser-cut lenses, with such added bells and whistles as light-sensitive self-tinting and antiglare coatings. Contact lenses have been around since the late 1800s and have been continually improved. With the advent of approved soft lenses that did not have to be removed at night in the 1980s, they gained increased popularity. Corrective laser surgery as an option became widely available in the 1990s, as did improved cataract surgery by laser. The associated implanting of artificial intraocular lenses has been popular since the 1960s. While a bionic eye exists in various forms, there's nothing that is implantable and functions like a normal eye. That will take time. What is closest on the horizon, perhaps available to you and me within ten years, is stem-cell (master cells that can be made to turn into other types of cells) regeneration of retinal ganglion cells that can repair blindness from glaucoma and related conditions.

Ears: Long gone are the days of the ear trumpet. Hearing aids keep getting smaller and smaller and better and better. That's good news, of course, because as we all know too well, hearing is sure to go—50 percent of people at age seventy-five have suffered some hearing loss—and the social consequences are not healthy. Many older people who suffer untreated hearing loss end up becoming increasingly isolated since they have too much trouble processing and interacting with the world around them. This can lead to loneliness and even depression. Hearing aids only make a sound louder. If the inner ear is damaged and the sensory cells do not function properly, then a cochlear implant is now often the solution. It is a neural prosthesis that creates "electronic hearing" by bypassing the damaged cells of the cochlea.

Heart: It's hardly possible anymore not to know someone who has had heart bypass surgery, which saved and prolonged his or her life. Since the 1960s, a growing number of people have had single, double, triple, and quadruple veins and arteries from elsewhere in the body grafted to the coronary arteries to improve circulation to the heart. Stents to reduce blockage and widen arteries are now very common and life extending. Diseased heart valves are also regularly repaired or replaced through surgery, using man-made materials or human or animal tissue. The biggest and rarest life-lengthening operation is, of course, a heart transplant, which has been available since 1967 to people with severe heart disease in imminent risk of dying, euphemistically called end-stage failure. About four thousand heart transplants take place annually worldwide, and on average fifteen years are added to a person's life with the operation. But it requires finding a healthy and compatible heart, and demand far exceeds supply. That has led to the development of mechanical or artificial hearts, usually as a bridge till a heart is found. Progress has been made since the 1980s, and in the past few years a series of portable heart pumps have been successfully employed, including at least one fully implantable one. A synthetic replacement heart is one of the top prizes of modern medicine, but it currently is beyond reach.

Other Organs: Kidneys are our most frequently transplanted organs today, followed by the liver. Transplantation medicine, unquestionably complex and challenging, continues to expand and evolve. Beyond heart, kidneys, and liver, lungs, intestines, pancreas, and thymus also are successfully transplanted today, as are various tissues such as tendons, veins, bones, and even corneas.

Our skin is both our largest organ and a tissue. Skin from one part of the body has long been grafted successfully to another part, most commonly in burn cases. But the future holds more promise in terms of both organ regeneration and synthetic skin with electrical neural-network sensitivity.

Teeth: Do you floss every day? Twice a day? It is one way to extend your life and to look good, really. Taking care of your teeth, like taking care of your skin, can make a huge difference in how well you look as you age. Flossing helps prevent gum disease, which if chronic can both cause your teeth to fall out and add plaque to your veins and arteries, thus increasing your chances of heart disease and a heart attack. My mother did not floss (Who had heard of it fifty years ago?), and while she taught me to brush my teeth, I cannot attest to what she did in private. But I know that like many people of her generation, her teeth and gums reached a point where the simple recommendation was to get all of the teeth pulled and get dentures. And that is how she lived for at least four decades...full plates of artificial teeth out at night and replaced in the morning. (She never quite accepted it, and it changed her smile!) Mankind has known false teeth for more than twenty-five hundred years. Full dentures have been around for about five hundred years, and porcelain teeth since 1770. Real progress, though, has come about in the last twenty-five years, meaning that for many, full plates of dentures are no longer necessary.

Partial dentures have also been around a long time, some removable, and others permanently fixed, such as crowns and bridges that are anchored to remaining teeth. They are more stable, of course, and technology has improved the look and feel of them.

With modern bonding techniques, teeth can be capped, veneered, and whitened, and these procedures, along with the replacement of missing teeth, all contribute to a better facial appearance and improved self-esteem. Modern techniques aided by computer modeling produce some fantastic results. Of course, false teeth that fill in gaps also contribute to clearer, more natural speech and enable one to chew and eat a variety of foods. So these are important replacement parts, not just to ensure proper function but to boost one's quality of health and chances for a long life.

For me, who once ran into an old-school dentist when I had a problem, and he willy-nilly suggested that I get a lot of my adjacent teeth pulled because they were eventually going to have problems and be extracted, I was saved by progress. The advances in dental techniques and technology have helped save my few problem teeth. For the two that could not be saved, two dental implants of the post-and-crown variety have been miracles of modern replacement medicine. That is real progress that enhances a long life. I only wish they were more affordable and available to more people.

Joints: Sports, arthritis, and nature's long-term wear and tear have resulted in massive numbers of joint-replacement procedures around the world. Hips, knees, ankles, elbows, and shoulders are commonly replaced successfully, relieving pain and increasing mobility. More than a million such replacements take place each year in the United States alone. While the body is often likened to a machine, it seems very much the case here since it is possible to head to the garage for a "tune-up" and a new part. Technology has been providing better and better parts in orthopedic prostheses. Artificial knees and hips last longer and work better.

TONY'S CASE

I have an acquaintance, Tony, who had both knees replaced— one in December and the other the following December. It took about six to eight weeks of postoperative recovery and physical therapy for him to be out and about and singing the praises of the operations. But one thing he found strange was that before he had the first operation, he had to shop for the knee he wanted. The surgeon and the second-opinion physician he consulted literally took out a parts catalog and went over the pros and cons of the various manufacturers' products. Before he made the final choice, he held the chosen part in his hands. The next year he assumed he would simply have the same artificial knee joint implanted in his other leg, but the parts catalog had new-and-improved models to choose from! Why put in last year's model that had been superseded— thanks to science and technology—by a better version? Today he is walking around well with two different artificial knees . . . and is proudly one inch taller.

Stem-Cell Regeneration: No question, a quantum leap in replacement and regenerative medicine has been the use and further potential use of stem cells (again, the master cells that can go into specialized cells) to replace or regenerate human tissues or organs. Someday, probably this century, you will be able to regrow an ear in a laboratory from your own cells. Lab-grown bladders already exist, and many more complex bioartificial organs are in the development pipeline. Even more approachable is the injection of stem cells or progenitor cells into parts of our bodies as seedlings to regenerate aging or failing organs.

If we are going to increase potential life expectancy to, say, 150, it will not only be because we can grow or regenerate more of the body's worn-out or damaged organs and tissues. (Currently the maximum potential life span is projected to be 125 to 130 years, though no fixed limit has or can be established.) It will also be because of bioengineered gene therapy, helping to make, for example, stronger knees or hearts by scientists altering DNA and creating naturally produced performance enhancements in our bodies through enzymes and proteins or by reengineering cells to provide protection and even immunity from various diseases. Corn today…a fresh brain tomorrow?

Brain: Sorry, no replacement part is available yet. But we now know that some brain cells have been shown to regenerate, something long thought impossible. And we do know that surgeons poking around inside our brains can achieve dramatic effects, such as calming the shaking associated with Parkinson's disease.

HOW OLD IS "AGED," OR SHOULD
I SAY "ELDERLY"?

So in the way the last generation used to think of sixty-five as being old, today many consider eighty as elderly. Thanks to science and technology, nutrition and exercise and lifestyle and medicines, the next generation may well think of ninety-five or one hundred as elderly . . . okay, *old*. France already has seventeen thousand *centenaires*, two-thirds women, and this one hundred–plus years category is growing fast.

Postadolescence, the two great killers around the world today are cancer and heart disease. And the two greatest drivers of greater longevity today are the improved awareness and treatment of these killers. According to the World Health Organization, 30 percent of cancers could be prevented. And happily, in my lifetime, recovery from breast cancer has improved tremendously, boosting life expectancies for women in most countries. Still, too many people die from breast cancer each year, especially in developing countries. While survival rates are high (over 80 percent) in Western countries, anything less than 100 percent is not acceptable, and we continue to look to science and medicine for more help. However, as early detection is a key to the best outcomes for all cancers, we need to first look to ourselves to avoid becoming a statistic.

Life expectancies will continue to increase over the coming years, with some estimates suggesting one hundred as the projected average life expectancy of Japanese women by 2050. You never know. The prospects of stem-cell regenerative organs, artificial organ implants, and reengineered DNA know no boundaries. Consequently, there are a growing number of people who pay to have their bodies "placed in cryonic suspension" (i.e., frozen), in hopes of being revived in a hundred or two hundred years, or whenever science has cures for what ailed them (including how to thaw their frozen bodies!).

Today, the challenge for most of us remains not living long, but living well. How do we increase our probabilities of enjoying extended, long, and healthy lives? Science and technology are on their way to making one hundred HLY (healthy life years) a reality.

12

LOVING, LAUGHING, WORKING

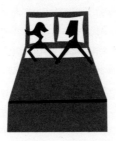

There are two things that save us in life, according to Indian journalist and novelist Tarun J. Tejpal: love and laughter. If you have one of the two, all is well. If you have both, you are invincible. Now there's an attitude.

I am not sure exactly when or how it began, but for more than a year now, I have awakened to e-mailed jokes and cartoons from French friends from around the world. It has caused me sometimes to break a personal rule: no e-mail before my morning routine and breakfast. The reason I've started this new routine is that I often laugh out loud from the jokes, and laughter is excellent medicine. Want to live longer?...Laugh a lot and often.

Study after study shows how laughter boosts one's mood, reduces blood pressure, increases circulation, and enhances one's immune system, even lowers bad cholesterol. So, laughter is right up there in my book with nature's "an apple a day keeps the doctor away." What's the worst thing that can happen if I read a joke or two before a cup of coffee? I die laughing?

I maintain—as I suspect most women do—a number of e-mail chains, and connections with personal, small social networks, which no doubt contribute to a healthier mental outlook for me than I would probably have without them. This small French joke group is a curious one. For starters, because it seems to pass through me, though I cannot tell a joke. I can tell a story, but I have never been one to remember or repeat joke after joke effectively. So, I have become a facilitator and communications hub, forwarding a joke from here to there and adding to the sidebar commentary. And depending on the joke, I may bring another person or two from my other networks into this cozy circle. It is curious because this group has self-selected into being all Francophones, all age forty-plus, and while broadly open in what we laugh at, we are very French in laughing about ourselves and laughing about aging.

I cannot claim the jokes are all brilliant (though some are), or that many are not silly (some certainly are). While many jokes are somewhat universal in appeal, others have a "you have to have been there" quality, which means you have to have been born and raised in France. Some are just shared takes on the absurdity of today's France or world. People have long recognized that the French approach to things can be arrogant and aggressive, voicing some opinions you may think but would not say in other cultures. But to the French there is a wry way to look at things with humor in mind, and nobody takes it seriously.

Putting on my "French" hat, I can also say the French tend to be the kind of people who, although we like to *râler* (grumble/be annoyed at all sorts of stuff because we love to have a discussion, i.e., "philosophize"), we don't like whiners and can't stand the kind of paralysis some people fall into because they are not happy with the choices they've made. We feel: "Get on, work on yourself." I promise you, some mornings I do sometimes laugh out loud so much that my sides ache and I have passed a daily aerobic fitness test.

Some notes are just grins and shrugs. I might wake to a line such as "When you are old, if you wake up without some pain...you are dead." Or "Age does not count, unless you are a (French) cheese" (that's one of those "you have to be French" jokes). Or the somewhat generic "It is impossible to give you my age, it changes all the time," or "Il est sur la liste rouge" (It's unlisted). I know these may not be great jokes, but they are humorous. "God did things well because as wrinkles increase, sight decreases."

In most cultures people laugh, publicly or covertly, about their politicians, bureaucracy, and government. France today is setting standards for petty bureaucracy and for tragic-comic politicians, so one would have to know the cast of characters and the language puns to appreciate the vicious humor that is the daily medicine that comes my way. The joke threads on aging require an appreciation for the French attitude toward aging. It is respectful and accepting.

Recently a Parisian friend in her late sixties sent a bunch of us (Frenchies) a text on aging that the French raconteur and philosopher Bernard Pivot had written, and the first response (we were all copied on it) came from her best friend (ten years younger) who said, "Magnifique...and by the way, hello, oldie."

I am sure she laughed when she read it. I did, and I am sure we all did, as we all know how hard she has worked to age...with attitude. It showed wit and respect. And another then responded: "Vivre c'est vieillir rien de plus," a line from Simone de Beauvoir (Living is aging, nothing more). And we were off being armchair philosophers, or rather simply being French. Except me, I saved that part for after breakfast.

Being French and being human, you can imagine the jokes and cartoons often have "content of a sexual nature." So I open up a cartoon of two giant turtles on a beach with the male saying to the female, "Let's have sex again," and the female replies, "So glad you asked, last time was 150 years ago."

Another participant shared a joke from the French humorist Guy Bedos, who at age fifty-nine said, "What consoles me about soon blowing my sixtieth candle is that in the word *sexagénaire* [sexagenarian] the word *sex* is included."

How do you keep humor in your life? As we age, humor is important both mentally and physically. It changes the look on our faces. ☺

SEX

I have now adroitly transitioned from the fact that laughter is good for aging to the inevitable topic of sex. Let us reaffirm what every publication that has an article championing aging well or with grace (how about with attitude, *s'il vous plaît?*) trumpets: a healthy sex life into old, old age improves health and can add years to one's life. Of course, the publications use more vivid language to express such ideas.

Sex as an anti-aging potion has both truth and appeal. Yes, orgasms reduce stress, help you sleep better, give your heart a good workout, help you live longer, help you live your time more richly. Adding supportive statistics here is almost comic. If you need them, they are there...including some biomedical explanations of why you feel better. And we're talking mostly sex, not love, in all its dimensions.

We have issues. How do we ignite sexual excitement in an old relationship? How do we deal with decreased sexual drive after menopause? How do we deal simply with sex once it becomes more difficult as we age? The simple answer is to acknowledge and deal with these issues because they are important. I wish here I could give you some big, juicy stories. But they are in the other book...the one I am *not* writing.

My friend Gaby took an expression by Jeanne Moreau and turned it into an expression I endorse: sex is like a potage— the first tablespoons are too hot, the last ones can be too cold, but we French enjoy a delicious vichyssoise (a cold soup) any time.

Sex should be integrated into our adult lives at any and every stage. It is important to create space for desire (when we are young we are tired, later we slow down, etc.). Ban the excuses and learn that sex, too, requires some preparation and shouldn't be relegated to mere leisure in mature life. Find ways to eroticize daily life and be a bit *coquin(e)* (mischievous).

The secretion of endorphins during sex puts one in a good mood and boosts efficiency (including at work!).

We certainly all have heard warm and fuzzy stories of a ninety-two-year-old woman marrying an eighty-seven-year-old man in some retirement village and boasting about their sex life. Good for them, and good for science, and good for Viagra sales.

I wish I knew what French men think about Viagra. I don't, and can't find a reliable answer. "Viagra, what's that? Ha-ha." French men consider sex a national institution they must protect. But Viagra is a game changer in our lifetime. I am sure it gives men the confidence to be tender, romantic, and sexual. More important, I believe it gives men the ability to continue to dream, to exercise and celebrate the imagination, to hope, and to enjoy life. Surely women and men benefit from that.

The way jokes weave their way into sex is interwoven with the power of relationships. And relationships as we age are the real deal to living well, aren't they?

ANCHORS

As a businesswoman who rose in a male-dominated industry, I was often asked to speak to women trying to balance business with life, without sacrificing too much of one for the other.

I told them I believed in four anchors, the sort of weights that hold down the shade canopies at the outdoor markets in

France or where I shop in Union Square in New York. These four weights keep us firm and balanced and sheltered: (1) good health; (2) a functional social network of friends and family; (3) a solid employment situation; and (4) time, space, rules, and practices for yourself. I said, "They work together, interacting in sometimes mysterious ways, and some stronger anchors can compensate for weaker ones, but the stress will become apparent then. Lose one of the anchors, and you are left twisting in the wind and out of balance."

As I contemplate aging with attitude, it is clear that jokes and sex are good for us, but (1) health is an anchor. Jokes and sex just contribute to the weight of that anchor. I have taken long passages in this book to offer my current approaches to and attitudes on embracing good health practices as we age. There's no doubt that (2) a functional social network of friends and family is an absolute necessity for quality of aged life, but the networks evolve with the times and surely are customized to the user. (3) Work or an activity we care about helps us fill our days with purpose (more on that later in this chapter). The idea of (4) time, space, principles, and policies for oneself is surely an anchor easier to understand, accept, and achieve in advancing years than in formative ones. These can range from taking the painting class you always wanted to, to watching some TV show religiously, or to keeping up your subscription to (fill in the blank, from magazines to season tickets to opera or professional sports, or a subscription to a gym, to a club, to...), or to taking the annual or semiannual vacation no matter what. Hair every Friday? Why not?

RELATIONSHIPS

Among the strongest anchors in life is, of course, a good marriage. Men have it a little better in this respect than women. Married men live longer than unmarried men. Not hard to figure out why. So, if you are keeping score, add a year or two to your mate's life expectancy.

As we know, women often outlive their husbands, or, in some cases, divorce them. While men do not handle divorce as well in terms of life expectancy as women do, women who are divorced live as long as those who are married. The key to a long, healthy, and contented life for a single woman is having fulfilling relationships. They are not the same as being or having been married, of course, but they are capable of providing what is needed to be healthy and happy.

People who are involved in meaningful relationships are healthier and thus live longer. How are your relationships? It is important to be connected, and that requires effort. Relationships need to be renewed and maintained, and new ones developed. Relationships with a spouse, with family members, and with friends of all kinds—and not to be glib, but even with pets—all have positive impacts.

If you want to live longer, develop your social network and relationships and see your stress reduced, your depression dissipate or never appear, and even your healthy behaviors increase. Friends certainly help you laugh. But you must work on developing and keeping your network. Pick up the phone, send a text or an e-mail. Be the one to organize a lunch. Present an occasion and environment where friends invite friends to meet you. Not only connect, but reconnect and grow.

Obviously, a spouse is logically one's best friend as one ages and one's most intimate friend. A spouse is the one who is there to provide encouragement, to help solve problems, little and big, to help keep one positive. And, as I have shared, maintaining a positive attitude adds healthy years.

LOVE, TENDERNESS, AFFECTION

The way environment is trumping genetics today, sometimes culture is a wild card in coming to terms with aging with attitude. Take love and sex. The attitudes are simply different in France than much of the world. *Vive la différence.* In a now celebrated study of older French and older Americans, it was revealed that 83 percent of the Americans felt that "true love can exist without a radiant sex life," while only 34 percent of the French believed it was possible. To me, this helps explain the French attitude of respect (held as a top value), longing, seduction, sensuality, and beauty as it relates to women of a certain age. And the study results speak to the power of imagination as a healthy component of aging with attitude.

However, there is, of course, more to love and a longtime relationship than sweaty sheets. I am often asked to explain my long, strong marriage. I've always been convinced that love, respect, trust, generosity, communication, tenderness, some common values, and a sense of humor are basic parts of a good relationship, but when it comes to ours, I'd accent that friendship, fidelity, and faith matter. And, on my part, a weird added element has been that I remain a bit intimidated by my man's superintelligence. Diane Vreeland wrote about the same sort of feeling in a relationship where she described herself as remaining "shy." I know it keeps me on my toes, adding a sense of mystery and surprise to the relationship and keeping the flame hot and going. We each have our differences, and a marriage of two cultures is certainly an extra challenge, but oh, so rewarding and rich.

I have a friend who has been married over thirty years and likes to say the key to a good marriage is having separate bathrooms. I rather think Helen Mirren, who turned a long relationship into a late marriage, has captured a more important key and thinks like me: "People get together for reasons other than sex, and although it's important for most couples, it's not what makes marriages last. I think the power of partnership in marriage is under-recognized in our society. That's what makes marriage work."

"Working" on aging with attitude certainly requires a "good" solitude, which is a spiritual and joyful one. It takes some inner searching to understand and appreciate that charm and emotions don't age, and we don't need to always talk or do stuff together to feel another's presence. Just being near a loved one can be a calming emotional reassurance. There is a tenderness associated with a long marriage and with a long life. Too often it's only the stuff of movies to see how one aging and very sick person takes care of the other through all sorts of hardships and negatives. But there can be years of healthy aging together these days if we work on some preventive schedule. Of course, poor health can become out of control, but...Loss goes with aging; however, it is not nearly as powerful or as traumatic as it is earlier in life. The loss of one's parents or a sibling or, horror of horrors, a child is nearly irreconcilable. If one lives to a grand old age, loss is an accepted part of life. It comes with the territory.

The healing power of touch also needs to be acknowledged as anti-aging medication. Touches, caresses, and kisses during a day make a difference. All things tactile seem to. Massages are good for one's circulation and cerebral calm, as is something as simple as stroking a pet. My sixty-five-year-old friend Danièle likes to say, "A half dozen physical touches a day are for maintenance; a dozen, well, that's something else, ha-ha."

In building networks of friends, it is worth noting that sometimes like-minded and aged friends are even more valuable in dealing with one's advanced years than family, at least in some cases. Here are people who can be counted upon and who can discuss the exigencies of age with experience and compassion. But while it is good to have aged peers in one's circle, I believe it is equally important to have a younger set of friends (beyond grandchildren). I have had several people tell me that having too many elderly friends is dulling, as too often age and health become repeat topics. I work at keeping younger people in my circle. Not only can one's learned lessons be shared with them, but they keep one current and thinking about the future. Younger people are positives in a world where positive thinking wins...at least it wins more quality time.

EMPLOYMENT

But what about the solid employment situation as anchor? I still believe in it. I am not comfortable with the stability of a three-legged stool in old age when our balance isn't what it used to be. A key, it seems to me, to attacking old age with attitude in post-work, retirement years is to "stay employed." That is, find some sustaining "employment," and not just playing out one's years. For perhaps a third or half of one's life, employment meant working for pay, or perhaps raising a family. It provided reasons to get up in the morning and for planning ahead and looking forward to some things.

Sure, some retirees build a comfort period based on the clocks and locations of their children, and especially grandchildren, but I wonder how sustainable and rewarding that is. If it works, fine, but I suspect for some it is an invitation to eventual pain and imbalance. It is also a reminder to build a broad network of relationships as part of your anchor.

I understand and admire those "retirees" who do not need to work anymore for the income (though I am sure a little extra is nice), but who choose to work the cash register or the aisles at a large store so as to be able to be with people, colleagues, and to have a schedule that reminds them that every day is not Saturday. It did not matter if they were a CEO or a salesperson; volunteering at the counter in a hospital or library or working the checkout line at a hardware store is fine. They already know who they are. That's the nice thing about advanced years.

Some people in today's economy simply need to work as long as they possibly can to financially maintain their homes and lives, so finding the employment anchor is only as hard as finding a job that is compatible with an individual's health, stamina, current skills, and mental outlook. Once they land on one, they tend to be happy campers. It is again about finding balance and being *bien dans sa peau*.

The way I saw the need to build this anchor for myself was by realizing life is built in episodes and stages. Episodes are short phases with discrete events or chapters that play out. Stages are bigger, inevitable, chronological....Childhood is a stage. So is retirement. What would I do after my job at LVMH and Clicquot? Some people never retire or semi-retire, like attorneys who keep an office into their nineties. That's one way to address the real need for a fourth leg to secure coverage.

I thought in terms of a third act. Perhaps I will need to come up with a fourth act? Why not? Shakespeare wrote the greatest plays in history in five acts.

ACT 3.5 *ENCORE MOI* (ME AGAIN)

Regardless of age, it's still vital to have our dreams. To keep dreaming is a way of shifting our focus to the "next" phase and stage of our impressive longevity; what we used to call the "third act" now has a fourth. Going from one phase to the next is not always easy—like a new freedom—so for many of us it is necessary to have some structure in our lives to avoid chaos and confusion. Many of us find a new vitality after forty or fifty or sixty, but don't always know how to channel it efficiently. The transition periods can be challenging because we must redefine ourselves and reset our priorities, and no one else can really do it for us.

My own "third act" is a case in point. I certainly never dreamed that one day I would become a writer or author. Actually, once I was well into it, I realized I did have that dream, though only for a few brief years, and only because my mother thought so and influenced me.

I was very good in my French writing class in high school simply because I had a fabulous teacher (I think I was in love with him and he knew it). He was neither good-looking nor young, but he was passionate about writing, reading, and literature (he had published a couple of novels) and had this amazing way of showing us how to look at a poem or a character in a book. I used to look forward to every class (one hour, five days a week). I grew tremendously in his class, and from then on loved literature more and more. *Perhaps someday I could write stories*, I had thought.

It was my father who gave me the basics, teaching me how to read and write when I was five and making me curious about other cultures via geography, learning (like many French kids, maybe it was a trick of the time) the capitals of the major countries and their places on a globe. Through my high school years, Mom would always declare that if she had had the same opportunity as a young girl, she'd work hard to get the only medal worth getting, *les arts et les lettres*, and was hoping that someday I'd get it. The praise I'd get for my "dissertations" (essays) made her say this, as compliments were rarely part of my educational support system. In any event, the "writing dream" was somehow put into a little box and forgotten about when I decided to study languages in Paris after my year in the United States as an exchange student.

Later I went into business, and although I had to write reports, press releases, and letters, I never thought about it as writing. It was only when in my fifties an agent got me a contract for *French Women Don't Get Fat*, and it became a success and a best seller, that the bell rang and the dream came back. I am sure many of us have similar stories about certain dreams we put aside, and then one day they pop up again. Like real estate, it's all about location and timing! For me, this meant changing jobs, as it was clear I could not manage doing my day job as a CEO and writing and promoting my book(s). I saw this as a signal and opportunity to move on. In a way, I like to say that my third act was handed to me on a silver platter. Working what seemed like part-time was enticing, so I could have time to play. It did not start quite that way.... It seemed I was working time and a half.

Was the transition easy? Yes and no. On the plus side, I did not have to go to an office anymore, nor work ten or more hours a day, attend lots of meetings, travel more than I liked, to places I often didn't care too much for, report to someone, or do many other chores that had to do with a corporate job that was part of the largest luxury group in the world. On the minus side, it was a bit more subtle: at first I did not have the time to think and analyze, but looking back, writing was demanding and draining, and along with that came traveling to promote the book, doing interviews, photo sessions, giving lectures, going on radio and TV, creating a website and maintaining it (and later doing the Facebook, Twitter, and other social media expected of a writer these days). Although all of it was thrilling, it was exhausting.

The insidious and painful part is that when the books launched, promotions and speeches took me away from home and friends much more than I cared for and gave me very little time for myself through my first four books. Yes, writing (it helps to have a contract with a due date) gets me up in the morning; yes, it keeps me thinking and dreaming; yes, it fills my calendar for months, even years at a time; but it is a different kind of "work, work, work." Ten hours in the office? For a writer, the job is life. Forget hours. One gets trapped at times into the "adrenaline state" of being an author: meeting one's readers and all the activity and some excitement and deadlines with press. Additionally, I had not yet learned how to say no well enough and took on more and more side projects until it was clear that I could no longer handle everything well. No time to pause, no time to ask oneself questions. It's funny what drives us to perform. We keep running till some signal indicates time out. I found myself tired, sometimes overwhelmed by all the work, and too often unfocused. Not a nice feeling. I think the technical term is "pooped."

Only after four books, when I was pressed on all sides to sign for the next two, did I decide on my own to enact a drastic step by taking the summer completely off to think of the next stage, but mostly to rest and restore. Act 3.5? I was exhausted physically and emotionally. My books are published in thirty-seven languages and many more countries, and there wasn't a spare moment without the questions and requests and opportunities and responsibilities associated with the books! (I am grateful and thankful, of course.) It seemed to me that yesterday I was in the corporate world, and yet today it was somehow four years later! Yes, I was enjoying myself immensely, but was also totally drained and numbed at times, and I knew it was time to reconsider.

That summer, I had the privilege of spending my time in our Provence home, and it was telling: for the first time I had no article, book, or report to write; no responsibility; no long hours; no travel. Time is indeed the greatest luxury. I had no agenda but to enjoy myself, spend time with my husband, and take care of those visiting us and do whatever pleased me. I had the freedom to be me. I always thought I had a great and rich life until that summer—the first time since graduate school that I'd had a whole summer off. Wonderful.

Years of life's experiences had given me a sense of freedom, security, and self-confidence like never before. I found that my new social life, notions of generosity, and goals added to my emotional stability and wisdom, and I experienced a great level of comfort and happiness. It was like childhood or adolescence but without its disabilities. Oh yes, one learns to live with one's limits, but that is true for many stages of life, especially after fifty. The best for me was learning to say no, no, and no to all sorts of things that I could never have said no to before, like having a meal with someone I did not care for, going to an event that did not thrill me, and so on. That summer was "my time" or "me time," and it felt wonderful. Yes, too much of a good thing is . . . "wonderful," as Mae West used to say.

I also tried to figure out what matters most in my life, what things I love, and establish an inner set of priorities for the various times of "play." My "me time" becomes more and more vital as it is a way to replenish and rejuvenate, and I feel I need it physically as I age. I need my figurative "beach time" (literal sometimes, too), and the long morning walks in the countryside, when all is still asleep, as my luxury moment to replenish—to find silence and inner peace. It's a kind of walking meditation facing the glorious Alpilles (little Alps), smelling jasmine and fruit bushes throughout the *chemins* (paths) of the village, and heading to the bakery (oh, that smell at seven thirty when the first batches of fresh bread are just out!). Those moments under the morning sun are moments that never become boring. Solitary biking is equally good for me, as one can travel the various bike routes from lavender fields to growing fields (we are in one of the top garden areas of France for vegetables and fruit trees and some bulls in between), to farms with sheep and goats, to a small road with a twelfth-century chapel, to lanes with a spring running alongside and paths under shaded narrow *chemins* where one feels like one is crossing paradise. These are pleasures that heighten my sense of connecting with nature in a different way than walking in a city does.

That September, when I returned to New York with its pulsing energy (which I feel as soon as I head to Manhattan from the airport), I immediately started to write this book.

I thought about it a lot, and I have thrown away as much of what I have written as I have saved.

An important takeaway from this is that renewed employment—a job, a calling—is an important anchor in living long and well, but it is a stage and has episodes. My third act as a writer now has moved to act 3.5. I have an audience I treasure and try to serve by sharing what I have learned. For the first two books I was a possessed writer. Now I am a writer in possession of her life. It is about finding and adjusting one's balance through the other anchors needed for a healthy life, and to adjusting to the uncertainties and opportunities life and nature throw at you as you accumulate years.

What work gets you up or will get you up in your post-retirement years? What's your fourth anchor? How can you make it work in your life both financially and logistically? I confess I was very fortunate in being handed my encore career, and not everyone can be a writer. However, everyone can find something else if they work at it and keep their eyes open and are honest with themselves (sorry, probably too late to be an actress or astronaut). I believe that. And while our first attempt may be misguided...so what? Try again.

One further note (and story) on the "employment" anchor. In the play chapter, I touted the value of hobbies and play. There are hobbies that also fill the "employment" function. Remember the times you enjoyed what you did at work and when it did not feel like work? Well, if you enjoy what you do for fun, why can't it be integrated into your life as your "employment," providing structure and accomplishments in your life? Especially when you have nothing to prove to anyone. Perhaps do volunteer work helping others; it is another proven anti-aging action.

I have friends in America and another set in France who have done precisely the same thing. They turned their passion for going to yard and antiques sales into a weekend business as dealers. Instead of visiting outdoor markets and fairs as consumers of moderately priced items anywhere from ten to one hundred years old, they eventually acquired a semispecialized inventory, continue with pleasure acquiring more of what they like and know about, and now sit on the other side of the booths as sellers. Their schedule is their own. From spring to fall, they choose fairs to participate in, sell a few items, make a few trips, make a little money, but get out and socialize with consumers and especially with like-minded friends in their little weekend fraternity.

When I was an exchange student near Boston, I lived with the family of a book editor. He had a little manual "hobby" he loved: he re-caned chairs. Whether they were from a neighbor's kitchen, or an antique dealer's inventory, or a garage sale, he slowly and masterfully "worked," repairing chair after chair, duly noting its number in his life's accomplishments. I think he charged people $25 a chair so it felt something like a professional engagement and people symbolically acknowledged its value and his skill. I am sure he enjoyed the pocket money, but the benefits he sought and found from his arts-and-crafts hobby were hardly financial. When he retired and moved to Albuquerque, New Mexico, his tools and "assignments" moved with him. I visited him there when he was in his nineties, and he was proud to show me the current chair he was bringing back to life. No doubt he was still charging $25 and smiling to himself. He lived to be one hundred, and when he passed, his numbered list of completed chairs was very long and his workshop was filled with yet-to-be-filled commissions.

RELIGION

One final comment on anchors and connections. Many people turn to or return to religion or religious organizations as part of the fabric of their elder network. This makes perfectly good sense and is filled with healthy positives. And those with a strong faith rarely feel alone. Faith as a constant cannot be overemphasized as raising the quality and tone of one's life through the decades.

I learned that in my early years when I taught Sunday school and did missions with my church to help people in eastern Europe. Today, my constant connection is through churches. I simply cannot pass a church without going inside. I have detoured my husband to churches, especially in France, Italy, Greece, and Turkey, but also all over the world to places of worship, mosques, Buddhist temples, and more. The frisson and high emotion I feel walking inside them is a wonder and a comfort, whether it is a large cathedral like Notre Dame in Paris, St. Peter's in Rome, or closer to my heart and life as in the cathedral in Reims, with its Smiling Angel, or the smaller ones, which I prefer. I am always moved by stained-glass windows. The small and very old churches in Provence are my favorites. Christmas Eve at the Abbaye of Sénanque outside Gordes, where the monks still deliver the Mass and chant in Latin, has an atmosphere and spiritual quality that are sustaining in their simple beauty.

Visiting places of worship, belonging to a group, especially one with regular, shared activities and events to look forward to, is clearly more social and healthier than remaining isolated for much of the time. Clubs are good. And belonging to a club or religious organization (I don't mean to suggest they are one in the same, but both offer the opportunity to connect with like-minded people) gives one a place and greater confidence. It is also safe to say that on the whole, people who belong to religious groups are caring people and will help to look after others in need. That helps, including in reducing anxiety.

Perhaps most significant is maintaining a positive attitude. Being optimistic and even thinking yourself young and fit, as I have pointed out repeatedly, is a proven key to adding good years to your life. What is more positive than a religious belief in life after death? Do you have a spiritual life? Do you have a group with which you share concerns and activities?

13

NOW WHAT?

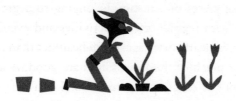

Peu à peu in practice means if you keep a list, you can add items to the list after you cross off the actions you've implemented. Personally, I collect a lot of ideas on scraps of paper, but eventually I simply need to sit down, sift through them, and create some simple order. It reminds me of the days we used to balance our checkbooks. I need a balanced checklist.

My ninety-four-year-old friend mentioned in the introduction has passed away. She was ready, and content with her life, and passed peacefully. When she was rushed to the hospital for her short, final stay, her nail polish was perfect. That's one measure of "If you have to go, that's the way to go." She had an amusing way with language and phrases that touched common sense with overtones of the universal and helped me to appreciate fundamentals. One phrase I have taken from her is "If I am alive in June, I'll worry about it then." She lived a lot of Junes, but in the last decades of her life she used the phrase to highlight the reality that the older we get, the more Zen-like living in the moment matters. It also points to a swing toward an overtly hedonistic philosophy, or as in another of her phrases, "What are you waiting for?"

That is one of the characteristics of aging with attitude, recalculating the trade-offs of future rewards (or securities) against relatively instant gratification, because "what are you waiting for?" It could be a vacation trip, cosmetic surgery, or buying that piece of jewelry you've always wanted. Seizing the moment for her as she increasingly lived with a mind that dropped the recent past meant enjoying the first corn on the cob of the season or a slice of carrot cake as if they were newly invented and a delight. They brought a spot of joy to her that was a pleasure to behold. She could sit in the country and look at the trees and flowers and sky with equal joy and contentment. She had no place to go, she would say. Another take on stopping to smell the roses.

But the correlation to broader bandwidth in life strikes me when I consider vacation or exotic travel. My friend built up memories that lasted her a lifetime. Lots from her early years and lots from her midlife extensive world travel— Wordsworthian "spots of time" that "retain a renovating virtue." It wasn't failed memory that made her later memories less vivid or meaningful; it was that the later experiences were more in and of the moment. I realize this now when I travel to a great new location or another new and great restaurant (after a life of eating at excellent restaurants); the experience and power are in the present tense. That's just the way it becomes. I live more in the present and for the moment. It is different but equal, as my friend taught me.

Just as important to aging with attitude is maintaining some inner eye on the future, an attitudinal and atmospheric retention and celebration of imagination in the old-fashioned sense of dreams and fancy. Bernard Pivot, reflecting on his becoming old, and having a young girl on a subway offer him her seat, put it this way: "To fight against aging is if at all possible not to renounce to anything. Not to work, not to travel, not to shows, not to books, not to *gourmandise*, not to love, not to sex, not to dream. To dream is to remember exquisite hours as much as we can. It's thinking about pretty dates that await us. It's letting one's mind idle between desire and utopia."

CATEGORICALLY YOURS

Olivier de Ladoucette, a French gerontologist, psychiatrist, and author, believes the French have three basic approaches to aging. His categories, if not his percentages, work for more than just the French and do help us to assess ourselves.

1. According to *Docteur* Ladoucette, 20 percent of the French are *gamblers*. These are the people who roll the dice with addictions and other harmful behaviors: smoking, being significantly overweight, abusing alcohol, et cetera. These are the people who don't want to

change their behavior, and claim, "You've got to die of something." It can't be easy being married or close to a gambler.

2. Fifty percent of the French are *mechanics*. They believe their bodies are something that can be fixed like a car. If you have high blood pressure, take pills, put an additive into your engine…no need to change your driving or lifestyle. Knee hurts? Exercise to build up muscles and range of motion? Nah, why try; just get a new knee. Of course, we all need a bit of a tune-up and the benefits of contemporary medicine and technology, but you know the type—more men than women in France—who want the magic potion and believe there is a fix for all that they or life has inflicted upon them.

3. Thirty percent, according to Ladoucette, are *gardeners*. This category is dominated by women (why am I not surprised?), who have the greatest chance of living the longest time. Why? Gardeners observe, listen to their bodies, anticipate, and act.

I love gardening. I like to do as much as I can myself, except boring things like mowing the lawn. Nowadays, I am reconciled to the fact that if I want pretty flowers and fruit, I must hire a professional to do some of the heavy lifting or to climb the ladders for the necessary pruning. And now and again, I need specialized expertise to identify and fight the diseases that crop up in my garden. I still do the weeding and the sweeping up. Same goes for how I approach my aging body.

And so now, I have written a gardening book (this book) with questions to help you tend your garden—yourself. If you do not like my little "mirror, mirror" conceit, I am sorry. It is the memory crutch and gimmick I use myself to assess and reassess who I really am now. The questions I ask directly or rhetorically or implicitly in the text are the questions it took me a lifetime to signify and value.

Here's my refresher checklist of about fifty simple and not-so-simple questions that range from holistic to tactical to big-picture, to some questioning whether to buy a new pair of shoes and with what size heel. I hope you will take time to stop and think, and jot down some notes. Perhaps respond to five or ten in the coming days and revisit the list again and again. Make plans, live long and well. For me, a crucial part of aging with attitude is to check in with myself frequently and to ask the right questions.

- What does my appearance say to people I meet?
- Do I look the best I can for my age?
- How do I feel about aging and myself?
- Do I have fulfilling relationships?
- What is in my control that can improve my health short- and long-term?
- Am I overdue for a physical examination? A dental examination?
- Does my clothing style suit my age and me?
- Has the time come to retire my bikini? And how about those high heels?

- How do I retain and adapt my style signatures in passing years?
- Do I wear sunglasses?
- Do I always wear sunscreen when I go outdoors?
- Did I moisturize today? Did I floss?
- How did I take care of my face this week?
- Why do I want a (or another) facelift?
- Do I have the right hairstyle for my face...for who I am today?
- Do I utilize the best treatments for my hair?
- Am I at peace with my hair color—should I color it or not?
- Have I built sufficient movement into my life at this stage?
- Just how much moderate exercise am I getting? The right exercises?
- Strength training? Balance fitness?
- How are my joints doing? What am I doing for them?
- What am I doing to maintain erect posture?
- Do I take the stairs? Take a walk daily?
- Have I adjusted my intake of food and alcohol for my current stage in life and level of activity?
- How do I give up diets? Why should I? What's wrong with diets?
- How do I reconcile my relationship with food?
- Is cooking at home so vital? If I eat out, how should I eat?
- Are vitamins and other supplements necessary?
- How much water is sufficient? What's the proper daily "dose"?

- How many food colors am I eating a day?
- Am I eating three meals a day? Am I skipping one meal and bingeing on another?
- Am I snacking between meals? Am I eating when I am not hungry?
- Do I have "offenders," foods or food practices that I should know with my head to control?
- Am I prepared for the postmenopause stage?
- Is estrogen in my equation?
- Is a calcium supplement good medicine for me?
- What gets me up in the morning? What will get me up in the morning in the years to come?
- Are my long-term finances in order?
- What will be my third act? What about act 3.5?
- Do I program some "me time" into every day? Am I overdue for a vacation?
- Do I have a spiritual life?
- Do I work at maintaining a circle of friends of various ages?
- Do I have a network of friends I can count on?
- Do I have a sex life?
- What are the rituals I follow in preparing for sleep?
- How many hours of sleep am I getting, and is it enough?
- Have I laughed today?
- What's my idea of play? Okay, what's my other idea of play?

WOMEN AGING WITH ATTITUDE

My friend Erin and I got to thinking about which women stand out as aging with one or more of the attitudes that I respect and espouse. We each know plenty of people personally whom we admire for doing this or that or looking or behaving just so; they are small-town heroes and role models. On the world's stage, we mostly find politicians and actors and perhaps a few sports or news celebrities. So we sent out an online questionnaire to a few hundred friends in hopes of getting some more prime examples of well-known women who inspire us.

They gave us a few ideas, and we did not get a host of stand-out French women. It seems Jeanne d'Arc, who lived six hundred years ago, did not enjoy a long life, dying at the stake at age nineteen. Now, Madame Clicquot, the "Widow" Clicquot (1777–1866), whose story I have told professionally hundreds of times and remains famous in France, sets a good example of aging with attitude, living long and well. Taking over her husband's small champagne business when he died suddenly in 1806, she became arguably the world's first modern businesswoman. Growing the business globally to renown, she was credited with both technical and commercial innovations that reshaped an industry. Her motto, "One quality...the finest," continues to infuse and distinguish the firm that still bears her name.

But she is long dead, too. Who today can we point to for insights into productive persistence?

Queen Elizabeth II of England has the longevity and the respect of almost everyone for a life of service to others. She gets up and goes to work seemingly every day, decade after decade. And I love that when she gets annoyed, she reportedly rotates her wedding band or says, "I am not amused." Plus, she still enjoys shortbread cookies.

Miuccia Prada shows her attitude by never wearing blue jeans (me neither) and for being different as an intellectual of fashion (while being one of the most influential designers in the world today). She is one who says that thinking about age all the time is the biggest prison women can make for themselves.

Catherine Deneuve is France. Not an easy crown to wear—from sex symbol to artist to lifestyle model to social icon and more—and through the decades and the stages of her long life and looks, she has worn it admirably (and still seductively). She is a great gardener, and acts like a grounded and normal person, even if she is closer to an ideal. Plus, she regularly checks in on her mother of one hundred–plus years.

Then there is **Sophia Loren**, the Italian movie star diva of the first rank from an era of silver screen the likes of which we won't see again. She still acts the star and when asked, "What is your *élixir de jeunesse*?" (youth potion), she replies, "My mother's DNA and forty minutes of exercises each morning without a trainer." Plus, I like that she confesses to be tempted by all the *dolce* (sweets) at parties but has learned balance and restraint so as not to have to watch her diet for a week. Should she indulge, I expect she practices the same recalculating and recasting over the next day that I do to maintain my equilibrium.

The American dream is alive and personified in **Sonia Sotomayor,** the first Hispanic American justice on the United States Supreme Court. Her life story is the stuff of legend: Spanish as her first language; alcoholic father from Puerto Rico who died when she was nine; and a somewhat remote mother, also from Puerto Rico, who was an orphan. Raised in housing projects in the Bronx, New York, and a type 1 diabetic from age seven, she rose through superb attitude, smarts, education, and hard, hard work to the pinnacle of the law profession. Her accomplishments and winning personality burst upon the broader consciousness of the world when in her mid-fifties she joined the Supreme Court in 2009. And in 2012–2013, her powerful, best-selling memoir of her life up to 1992 brought her inspirational story to a broader public.

Tao Porchon surely has attitude, considering herself "just your average New York yoga instructor" six years before reaching the magic centenarian level, yet saying, "I'm going to dance and do yoga as long as I live."

The postmodern American dancer and choreographer **Trisha Brown** (adored by the French) is a master of movement and collaboration demonstrated through the decades. That she danced in her mid-seventies and choreographed till age seventy-six is impressive, but what is more impressive is that in her pursuit of pure movement and fluidity, she has remained true to her art while reinterpreting herself and her solo dances for her age and with her long-lived Trisha Brown Dance Company.

The woman mentioned most frequently in my little survey as aging admirably with attitude and style is **Hillary Clinton**. Whether you love her politics or not, it is clear she is a respected world figure who is the first woman in history to be accepted on her merits as a creditable candidate for president of the United States. She has lived her dramatic life in public with dignity and has displayed an extraordinary work ethic in the public service sector for decades.

Among women in politics, Germany's no-nonsense **Angela Merkel** has also stood out among men and women with her firm leadership and firmer ideas that have set a tone and skill set for Europe and for a new generation of leaders.

Michelle Obama is recognized for her brilliant education and educational values, her toned arms, her family values and priorities, her White House garden, and her vision and work to change America's eating habits. And, who knew, for her fashion influence? At the second Obama inauguration, her clothes and what designer she would choose sustained ongoing coverage.

How not to mention **Meryl Streep**? Catherine Deneuve admires her above all others for what she has achieved as the actress of her generation. Her unequaled linguistic and acting talents only hint at what has made her one of the busiest of actresses, even today in her sixties. And not only working and maturing in a range of adult roles that set a new standard and model for actresses and box offices, but consistently doing so with a dignity and style, an aplomb, that has further set her apart as exceptional.

I also admire the sometimes blonde, sometimes gray-haired **Helen Mirren** for carrying her sensual screen persona into her late sixties while at the same time putting her indelible stamp on queenly performances. Plus, at age sixty-seven she was named "Body of the Year." That's aging well—and add that to her style and other accomplishments. She lived an indulgent artist's life early on and married at the tender age of fifty-three, and enjoys dressing up rather than dressing down...all the time wearing a tattoo of a star on her left hand.

There are no Coco Chanels today; perhaps there can no longer be transformative designers, only brands, so I celebrate passionate, independent designers such as **Béatrice Ferrant**, a quintessential woman designer on the Paris fashion scene with a very special sense of style built on vast knowledge and technique. Her small boutique in the 6ème has but a few pieces, all of sheer beauty and with a less-is-more kind of style. Less is more equals my kind of aging with attitude.

Zaha Hadid is the first woman to win the top honor in the field of architecture, the Pritzker Architecture Prize. She's known for being different, defying convention, and seemingly not following any rule, including gravity.

Yoko Ono stands long and tall for a short woman who has dealt with character bashing, kidnapping, deportation, and assassination, all in public view. Time has vindicated and validated her, and she has aged well by not changing. She has been described as the ultimate feminist who does not need us to like her. She simply does not care what we think about her as a woman. Her purpose is to try to free people in what she does in art and by telling the naked truth.

It certainly is impossible not to be impressed by **Aung San Suu Kyi** for her lifelong fight for democracy in Burma, now Myanmar. Of course, a great natural beauty into her sixties, winning the Nobel Peace Prize, and a major film of her life helped bring to the forefront her strengths and struggles.

Jeanne Moreau is *un personnage* (a character) and one of France's most accomplished actresses as well as a singer and director. Post-eighty-five she is still at it, opining regularly and saying smart and provocative things, acting, and, alas, still smoking (I suppose one should look the other way for someone of her vintage). She has aged with style and attitude *à la française*. To my generation, she is best remembered for her part in *Jules et Jim*, but she has been featured in over fifty films and built a body of work (1949–2012) that is unsurpassed. In the 2012 *Une Estonienne à Paris* (*A Lady in Paris*), an elegant comedy drama, her sheer charisma reminds us that female beauty is ageless.

My most heartfelt recognition probably goes to my young-est friend—no, not my boyfriend of the *Ouverture*, but three-year-old **Simone**, the young French lady who has yet to eat processed food and started to learn to cook at three years of age. This past Christmas, she wrote her first letter to Santa. Her number one item on her Christmas list? Scotch tape. And when she ran into Santa Claus at the local town hall, she did not hesitate to ask if he had gotten her letter and "will I get the Scotch tape?" The characteristically French Santa replied, "Yes, *la mère Noël* (Mrs. Claus) is taking care of it." Simone was delighted. Her blend of pragmatism and fancy should serve her well and long.

In the final and famous line of Voltaire's most celebrated work, Candide says, "Il faut cultiver son jardin" (We must cul-tivate our garden). Here Candide is for the most part rejecting Pangloss's utopian optimism for pragmatism. He got it half right, whereas Simone has got it all right. We need optimism and pragmatism; a positive, progressive attitude; and a realis-tic plan to grow our gardens well over the years.

Voltaire, a practiced gardener himself in life and philoso-phy, knew as much. He knew that gardens are about dreams and imagination, but to produce an aesthetically pleasing outcome requires planning, care, and especially weeding. In many ways, a mature garden requires more effort and cultivation than a young one. Coaxing nature each year to show its best is about anticipation, hope, luck, and optimism. Cultivating one's garden is about essential pragmatism with an attitude that is realistic yet positive and aspiring. Simone has indeed got it right. (And she got the Scotch tape.)

Happy gardening. *Bonne chance et bonne santé.*

Leek Detox

This is the recipe for the French weekend leek detox, mentioned on p. 135.

SERVES 1

1kg (2lb) leeks
Water to cover
Salt and freshly ground pepper, and parsley to garnish

1. Clean the leeks and rinse well to get rid of sand and soil. Cut off the dark-green parts, leaving all the white parts plus a suggestion of pale green. (Reserve the extra greens for soup stock.)
2. Put the leeks in a large pot and cover with water. Bring to the boil, reduce the heat, and simmer uncovered for 20–30 minutes.
3. Pour off the liquid and reserve. Place the leeks in a bowl. Season sparingly with salt and pepper, and garnish with parsley if you wish.

REMERCIEMENTS

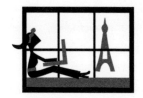

French women don't...write books without help from friends. This book is filled with advice and stories I have absorbed from many friends, some of whom are named in the text with their real names and some somewhat disguised with new names to protect them from my liberties. Thank you, dear friends—those named, referenced, and unnamed—and I count on you in the days ahead.

My agent, Kathy Robbins, merits a great deal of credit for making this book happen. One day she said, to my astonishment, "*French Women Don't Get Facelifts* should be your next book." And she kept at it until I agreed, thus leaving me with a title and a book contract and a couple of years to fill in the content. She believed that my helpful take on aging, told in my way, is what my readers and many new ones would enjoy and benefit from. Hopefully that's true. If not, blame her for the title and me for the rest. I am, in fact, blessed with readers who encouraged me to write this book and whose lives touch mine in so many ways. *Merci*.

Over the course of writing my books, I have been fortunate

to develop a team I respect and can count on. R. "Nick" Nichols has supplied his wit and wonderful illustrations to all my books and given them a visual identity I very much appreciate and enjoy. Erin Jones Eichenstein has again helped with the manuscript, reading early drafts and offering suggestions, adding facts and making improvements, and providing encouragement. So, too, has Sarah Hearn Morrison, who beyond being an early reader of the text returned as the recipe tester and caught bits of Franglais cooking that would have missed the mark both in France and America. Thanks again, Erin and Sarah, both of whom got married between my last book and this one!

Newest to the team is Karen Murgolo, VP, Editorial Director of Grand Central Life & Style, my editor for this and my next book. She has proven to be the best of editors to me: organized, efficient, proactive, timely, and helpful without being intrusive or burdensome. I appreciate her support, encouragement, and expertise.

My husband, Edward, has had to live with this book almost daily for a few years, and that he is still smiling and talking to me is a small miracle of love. All too often, especially at breakfast and dinner, I would get carried away telling him my latest ideas and musings and information for the book and continue with political opinions and philosophizing to the point where he would say, "Interesting, but what does that have to do with aging with attitude?" The book is better for his counsel. And my life is better and richer for having him as my sidekick in attempting to age with style and attitude.

INDEX

ABOUT THE AUTHOR

Mireille Guiliano is the author of the international bestseller *French Women Don't Get Fat*. A former chief executive at Louis Vuitton Moët Hennessy (LVMH), Mireille is 'the high priestess of French lady wisdom' (*USA Today*) and 'ambassador of France and its art of living' (*Le Figaro*). She is a frequent public speaker – nationally and internationally – on business topics, especially related to the luxury-goods sector, as well as on wine, gastronomy and lifestyle. Mireille has appeared on *The Today Show* and *Oprah* and has been profiled in *The New York Times*, *USA Today*, *Time*, *Newsweek*, *People*, *Business Week*, *Travel & Leisure*, *Food & Wine* and many more. Born in France, Mireille now divides her time between New York, Paris and Provence.

www.mireilleguiliano.com